OXFORD
UNIVERSITY PRESS

Oxford University Press, Inc., publishes works that further
Oxford University's objective of excellence
in research, scholarship, and education.

Oxford   New York
Auckland   Cape Town   Dar es Salaam   Hong Kong   Karachi
Kuala Lumpur   Madrid   Melbourne   Mexico City   Nairobi
New Delhi   Shanghai   Taipei   Toronto

With offices in
Argentina   Austria   Brazil   Chile   Czech Republic   France   Greece
Guatemala   Hungary   Italy   Japan   Poland   Portugal   Singapore
South Korea   Switzerland   Thailand   Turkey   Ukraine   Vietnam

Copyright © 2010 by Oxford University Press, Inc.

Published by Oxford University Press, Inc.
198 Madison Avenue, New York, New York 10016
www.oup.com

Library of Congress Cataloging-in-Publication Data

Zorumski, Charles F.
Demystifying psychiatry : a resource for patients and families / Charles F. Zorumski and Eugene H. Rubin.
p. cm.
Includes bibliographical references and index.
ISBN 978-0-19-538640-0
1. Psychiatry—Popular works. I. Rubin, Eugene H. II. Title.
RC460.Z96 2009
616.89—dc22   2009010336

Printed in USA
on acid-free paper

Contents

Preface

Psychiatry is pseudoscience. You don't know the history of psychiatry. I do.
—Tom Cruise, Actor, 2005

Psychiatry is arguably the most misunderstood specialty in modern medicine. A great deal of mystique and myth surrounds this clinical discipline. There is an impression that psychiatrists are part physician, part confessor, part police officer, and part shaman. In a way, psychiatry is similar to the fields of philosophy and politics: Everyone, regardless of background, seems to have a strong opinion about the field. The problem is that only a limited number of people actually understand the discipline of psychiatry. Even many nonpsychiatric physicians have only a limited understanding of what psychiatry is or what psychiatrists actually do, and some peculiar and unfortunate behaviors on the part of some psychiatrists and other mental health professionals admittedly have contributed to this misunderstanding. Furthermore, some of the field's tendency to hold to archaic ways of thinking about the diagnosis and treatment of psychiatric disorders sometimes compounds the problem.

The purpose of this book is to offer a straightforward description of the field of psychiatry and of what general psychiatrists actually do, focusing on mental disorders that occur primarily in older adolescents and adults. The book is meant for nonmedical audiences, including patients and their families. We try to minimize (or at least explain) some of the jargon and technical terms used in the field. We also hope, however, that the book is useful for medical professionals as well as for psychiatrists and other mental health professionals. In fact, a lot of what we discuss in this book is taken from our efforts to teach our own medical students and psychiatry residents about the field, including its strengths and limitations and its importance as a research-based medical discipline.

At the outset, we should give the disclaimer that our view of psychiatry is heavily biased by our years at Washington University in St. Louis-School of Medicine. Washington University holds a somewhat unique place in American psychiatry. Beginning in the 1950s, and as a result of the efforts of several key individuals, including Eli Robins, Sam Guze, George Winokur, and Lee Robins, our department has championed a "medical model" approach to psychiatry. The department is driven by its commitment to research, and its core beliefs build on applying the medical model to psychiatric disorders. Rigorous data—not opinion and not mysticism—drive our work and clinical practice. In its simplest form, the medical model refers to an effort to diagnose, treat, and study psychiatric disorders using the same principles that have guided the tremendous successes in other fields of medicine. For us, this means a heavy emphasis on defining and refining the criteria used to diagnose psychiatric disorders as well as on understanding the long-term clinical course of the disorders, the means by which treatments influence the short- and long-term course, the genetic influences on psychiatric disorders, and ultimately the underlying neurobiology that produces these complex and at times devastating illnesses. The hope is that this approach will lead to better and more effective treatments.

Importantly, the medical model approach requires significant and meaningful interactions between patients and their physicians, interactions that are at the heart of all good medical care. The approach does not rely strictly on medications as the only or even the predominant form of treatment, but rather it emphasizes the importance of the doctor–patient relationship and a balanced approach to clinical care in working toward optimal outcomes. Thus, how psychiatrists interact with their patients as human beings is a critical part of clinical practice. Additionally, psychiatrists are only one component of the mental health care system, and we try to point out the important roles of a variety of other professionals, including psychologists, social workers, and counselors, in helping patients and their families to achieve the best results. We will repeatedly emphasize that the doctor–patient relationship and the involvement of a variety of professionals in clinical care are not unique to psychiatry but are components of all good medical care. In this respect, good clinical care in psychiatry is no different than good clinical care in any field of medicine.

As a result of great scientific and clinical advances and a shrouding in mystique, modern medicine has been elevated to a position of great respect in society. Doctors are generally held in high esteem and are rewarded with significant monetary compensation and accolades from grateful patients. Although much of modern medicine remains as much "art" as "science," particularly when it comes to treating common disorders like hypertension (high blood pressure), diabetes, and cancer, the public expects that medicine can fix all that ails us—that, in effect, there is a pill or a procedure for every problem. This is far from the truth. Even in areas where science lags tremendously, respect for physicians and the expectation that medicine can fix everything drive patients to accept a host of interventions that are of marginal benefit at best and may be harmful at worst. Examples include the common practice of prescribing antibiotics (e.g., penicillin-type drugs) for routine sore throats. The great majority of sore throats are caused by viruses, and the antibiotics do nothing other than to reassure the patient that a concerned professional is trying to do something to help. In fact, overprescription of antibiotics has adverse consequences leading to increasing strains of antibiotic-resistant bacteria. Similarly, ill-described disorders, such as fibromyalgia and reflex sympathetic dystrophy, sound medically impressive when diagnosed by a doctor, but they are often meaningless labels from a pathological perspective: Respectively, they simply mean widespread pain and intense pain out of proportion to the severity of the physical findings or injury. Nonetheless, these disorders receive aggressive and at times unfortunate and misguided treatments that have nothing to do with any identified underlying cause.

Psychiatry is not immune to these problems, and at times poorly conceived ideas have led to major problems for patients and their families. The unfortunate overuse of psychosurgical procedures ("lobotomies") in the early part of the 20th century, misguided psychological theories about the origins of schizophrenia and autism (that they're caused, for example, by the so-called "schizophrenogenic" or "refrigerator" mother), as well as the debacle resulting from psychotherapist-induced "recovered memories" are but three regrettable examples. In each of these examples, patients and their families suffered the consequences of bad logic and inappropriate "treatments." Despite these problems, medicine generally and psychiatry specifically have made great advances. Diagnoses are now much more reliably made, and treatments, while imperfect, are better than ever in terms of efficacy and side effects.

Our goal in this book is both to examine the current status of the field—including, where appropriate, the problems that it confronts—and to share our optimism for its future. Major advances in genetics and neuroscience now position psychiatry for rapid and amazing changes—advances that are likely to lead to novel techniques of diagnosis and treatment over the next several decades. Potential cures that were once thought unreachable for such devastating illnesses as Alzheimer's disease are now clearly within sight. Extensions of this type of progress to such psychiatric disorders as schizophrenia, bipolar disorder, and major depression are possible as well.

Many outstanding scientists and clinicians from around the world have contributed to the current state of psychiatry and the advances in the field. Because we are writing for nonscientists and nonclinicians, however, we have not tried to be comprehensive in our citations. We acknowledge at the outset that there are many colleagues and scientists whom we fail to mention, but whose work has been of major importance. We have selected a group of publications that we think will help readers to develop a better understanding of our rapidly developing field. Our bibliography includes a variety of books that have been written by outstanding scientists and clinicians for lay audiences. We emphasize these books because they provide insights into current thinking in clear and cogent ways, and we have found them helpful in shaping our own thinking and teaching.

Charles F. Zorumski, MD
Eugene H. Rubin, MD, PhD

Acknowledgments

Over the years, numerous colleagues have influenced our thinking about psychiatry and neuroscience. Several individuals—the late Eli Robins, Sam Guze, and Leonard Berg—mentored us during formative stages of our careers. All were highly inspirational individuals who significantly helped shape our thinking. Other key mentors include Gerry Fischbach and John Olney, as well as many colleagues and collaborators, including David Clifford, John Morris, Gene Johnson, Steve Mennerick, Doug Covey, and Yuki Izumi. We also feel privileged to be members of the Department of Psychiatry at Washington University in St. Louis. Our department has an extremely creative and collaborative environment, and our colleagues on the faculty have greatly influenced us over the years. While too numerous to mention by name, their constant interactions with us in our corridors, conferences, and seminars have sharpened our thinking about the field.

We are deeply indebted to the National Institutes of Health (NIH), particularly the National Institutes of Mental Health, Alcohol Abuse and Alcoholism, General Medical Sciences, and Aging, for their research funding. Without NIH support, there would be very little biomedical research, and creative thinking would be markedly curtailed. We also appreciate the ongoing support and friendship of Tom and Cherie Bantly and the Bantly Foundation. In addition, we have benefited from our interactions with the Alzheimer's Disease Research Center at Washington University.

In writing this book, we leaned heavily on numerous people for their opinions and critical comments. We are grateful to the team at Oxford University Press, including Yvonne Honigsberg, Marion Osmun, Craig Panner, and Shelley Reinhardt for their expertise and spirit of collaboration. We also benefited greatly from the input and support of our families, including Teresa, Erik, and Ian Zorumski, Donna Corno, and Dan and Beth Rubin. They not only provided continuous sources of encouragement but also read and critiqued various drafts of the manuscript. We are particularly indebted to Gene's wife and colleague, Dottie Kinscherf, for her devotion to this project. Dottie took on the herculean task of carefully reading, critiquing, and helping us to write and rewrite the entire manuscript. Without her efforts, this project would never have come to fruition.

Finally, we are profoundly indebted to our patients as well as the numerous psychiatric residents and medical students at Washington University. Our interactions with them were among our greatest influences and inspirations.

Demystifying Psychiatry

··· *one* ···

What Is Psychiatry?

Psychiatric disorders are among the most common maladies affecting humans. Current estimates indicate that at least one in three individuals has a diagnosable psychiatric disorder at some point in his or her life. Based on how frequently they occur in the population, psychiatric disorders are a bit like the common cold, although their symptoms and complications are much more devastating. Many psychiatric disorders go unrecognized and untreated, resulting in great costs in terms of suffering and lost productivity. To some extent, the under-recognition and undertreatment of psychiatric disorders reflect cultural biases against these disorders and a general misunderstanding of what the field of psychiatry is all about. In this chapter, we will discuss general aspects of psychiatry and set the stage for more specific discussions in later chapters about psychiatric disorders, their treatments, and their outcomes.

Psychiatry Is a Branch of Medicine

As a starting point, it is important to define what psychiatry is. Perhaps the simplest definition is that psychiatry is the medical specialty that deals with disorders affecting the human mind and behavior. This definition has two important components. First, psychiatrists are medical specialists, that is, physicians. They attend medical school and train in hospital settings just like other medical specialists, neurologists, and surgeons. Psychiatrists are taught to think about mental disorders as medical conditions resulting from altered brain function. By virtue of their training as physicians, psychiatrists are different from psychologists, social workers, or counselors, although the skills of all of these mental health professionals can be critical for helping patients to achieve optimal outcomes. Thus, in usual clinical practice settings, psychiatrists work closely with these other mental health professionals and form mental health delivery teams. However, only psychiatrists have in-depth training in human physiology, pathophysiology, medicine, and pharmacology and thus are the only mental health professionals allowed to order medical tests and procedures and, in most jurisdictions, to prescribe medications.

The second important aspect of our definition of psychiatry states that the specialty is concerned with abnormalities of the human mind and behavior. What do we mean by the term *human mind*? This is a problem that has vexed philosophers and scientists for millennia, but for our purposes we will use the fairly straightforward definition used today by leading neuroscientists. For these neuroscientists, the "mind" represents a set of integrated brain systems that allow human beings to do three important things—think; attach meaning to things, people, and events; and pursue goals. In the words of Joseph LeDoux, one of the leaders in this field, these three components form a "mental trilogy" and reflect brain systems underlying cognition (thinking), emotions (meaning), and motivation (goals).

Psychiatric disorders can be understood in terms of dysfunction in these three realms. For example, individuals with schizophrenia, a devastating and chronic illness characterized by hallucinations (false sensory perceptions) and delusions (fixed false beliefs that are out of context with the person's culture), show marked problems in thinking, memory, and problem solving. In fact, these "cognitive" symptoms contribute greatly to the disability associated with schizophrenia and are the reasons why it is difficult for these individuals to work or function in society. Additionally, patients with schizophrenia show marked problems with their emotions (referred to as "blunted" or "inappropriate" emotions) and have major defects in motivation. Similarly, patients with major depression not only have persistent problems with emotion (sadness), but they also show marked defects in thinking (particularly in the ability to focus and concentrate on a problem) and in motivation (interest in things around them). Treatment of these disorders attempts to improve all of these spheres, although achieving success across the three dimensions of the mind is a major clinical challenge.

Myths and Realities about Psychiatry

There are a lot of misconceptions about psychiatry. For this part of the discussion, we will borrow heavily from concepts previously put forward by Kevin Black and the late Sam Guze (pronounced Guzé), psychiatrists from Washington University in St. Louis. As they describe in *Washington University Adult Psychiatry*, one of the most prevalent myths about psychiatry is that "psychiatric illnesses aren't real." The corollary to this is that psychiatric disorders are really "problems of living" and thus don't require the attention of physicians. Sadly, it is true that psychiatric disorders are indeed "problems of living," but all serious medical disorders, such as cancer, heart disease, stroke, and diabetes, are "problems of living," and they cause people to seek help from physicians. The same is true for such illnesses as schizophrenia, bipolar disorder, dementia, and depression: They too cause people to seek medical care because physicians can help. Hence the concept of "problems of living" does not distinguish psychiatric disorders from medical disorders.

A second common myth, according to Black and Guze, evolves from a truism—that "psychiatry is an inexact science." It is indeed inexact, but this fact does not undermine its value as a field. Despite major advances in technology and science, much of modern medicine remains an inexact science. Psychiatry happens to deal with an area that is extremely complex to study, having to do with the aspects of our selves that make us most human. Great strides are being made in understanding the biology of the mind and mental disorders, but the state of the art is just that—a lot of art with an evolving science. Nonetheless, individuals suffer from psychiatric disorders, and their treatment must be done on the basis of incomplete understanding.

A third myth referred to by Black and Guze is that psychiatric diagnoses are meaningless labels because "even psychiatrists can't agree on diagnosis." This myth was actually true until around the 1960s. Then, in the latter part of the twentieth century, great progress was made in defining reliable criteria for psychiatric disorders. This work was driven in large part by an intrepid group of psychiatrists led by Eli Robins and Sam Guze at Washington University in St. Louis. Their efforts and those of numerous others resulted in a diagnostic system that, while still imperfect, is highly reliable, meaning that there is now excellent agreement among psychiatrists about the diagnosis in the majority of patients. The reliability of psychiatric diagnoses is as good as or better than the reliability of diagnoses in other branches of medicine. Some evidence indicates that the inter-rater reliability for major psychiatric diagnoses (e.g., schizophrenia, alcoholism, and major depression) is more than 80 to 90%—in other words, a very high degree of diagnostic agreement among doctors. This degree of agreement is rarely exceeded in any other branch of medicine, including in the interpretation of electrocardiograms (measures of heart electrical activity) or x-rays. What is less clear is how to establish the validity of these diagnoses. By validity, we mean the ability of a specific diagnosis to reflect specific underlying brain pathology (abnormalities of structure) or pathophysiology (abnormalities of function). Reliability and validity are separate descriptions of diagnosis and are somewhat independent; for example, some diagnoses can be highly reliable but have limited or no validity. We will attempt to deal with the challenges surrounding diagnostic validity later in this book.

A fourth myth is one that is actually perpetrated largely by psychiatrists when asked about the causes of psychiatric disorders. This is the myth of "chemical imbalance." As we discuss in Chapter 6, the mechanisms underlying psychiatric disorders are complex and poorly understood. The term *chemical imbalance* really just means that we don't actually know the cause, but based on the effects of medications, we have ways to improve at least some of the symptoms. This myth also shortchanges the importance of psychotherapy ("talk therapy") in helping patients to overcome their psychiatric disorders. The great hope is that this myth will cease to exist with advances in neuroscience and genetics and that the role of drug treatments and talk therapies will be much better understood.

Psychiatric Disorders and Public Health

When considering the statement that "psychiatric disorders aren't real," it is important to think about the problems that exist for individuals and society because of psychiatric illnesses. In 2004, public health scientists Mokdad and colleagues described the leading causes of death in the United States. At the top of the list were the usual suspects—heart disease, cancers, strokes, and lung disorders, in that order. These authors pursued this result further by asking a fairly simple but important question: What are the critical factors underlying these disorders? What they found was amazing from a psychiatric perspective. The three leading "causes" of death were actually tobacco use, poor diet and physical inactivity, and alcohol consumption, in that order. Other causes of death in the top ten included automobile accidents, firearms, risky sexual behaviors, and illicit drug use. Disorders involving drug use (including both legal drugs like nicotine and alcohol and illegal drugs like marijuana, cocaine, and heroin) are clearly psychiatric disorders and reflect disorders of the "mind." All drugs of abuse jump start and hijack reward and motivation systems in the brain. This is how these drugs are addicting. Similarly, about half of all car accidents and homicides involve the use of alcohol or other drugs, making these "psychiatrically related" as well. All told, nicotine and alcohol use and abuse were associated with more than 500,000 deaths in the United States in the year 2000. Problems associated with physical inactivity and poor diet (obesity) are complex but can reflect underlying psychiatric disorders and disruption of motivated behavior. Thus, at least some of the individuals with this risk factor are likely to have psychiatric disorders as well.

Another way to look at complications associated with psychiatric disorders is to ask how much these disorders cost the US and world economies. Data published in 2001 indicate that substance abuse disorders cost the US economy about $240 billion per year. By 2004, this figure had about doubled to more than $400 billion per year. By far, the leading drivers underlying these costs were alcoholism and nicotine dependence—two legal drugs. Other disorders in the top ten in terms of cost included Alzheimer's disease (#2), chronic pain (#3), depression (#4), and schizophrenia (#6). All of these disorders fall under the umbrella of psychiatry.

The costs of psychiatric disorders reflect both health care costs and disability or lost income. In the United States and Western Europe, about one in five persons has a disabling medical condition, meaning that they are unable to hold productive employment because of their illness. Mental disorders, alcohol and drug dependence, and Alzheimer's disease (in that order) are the three leading causes of disability, reflecting almost half of all disabling illnesses in western economies. A key question is why psychiatric disorders cost so much. Again, this is a complex issue but likely reflects the fact that the disorders are common (e.g., depression affects about 1 in 5 of the population lifetime), can be severe (resulting in suicide and premature death in the case of substance abuse, depression, and schizophrenia), and cause absenteeism from work and lost productivity while at work. It is estimated that persons who are seriously ill with major psychiatric disorders (e.g., major depression and alcoholism) miss more than two months of work per year due to their illness. Even moderately ill persons miss about two weeks of work per year. Persons with depression who try to go to work also experience lost productivity, costing them about six hours per week on average during the time they are depressed. A final factor that contributes to the costs is that psychiatric disorders, particularly depression, often occur in the presence of other medical conditions, such as heart disease, diabetes, and cancer. Having depression worsens the outcome of these medical disorders, which in turn worsen the outcome of depression, resulting in a negative double whammy on the individual.

Prevalence and Treatment of Psychiatric Disorders

Just how common are psychiatric disorders in the United States? A recent major study called the National Comorbidity Study-Replication (NCS-R), comparing data from1990 to 1992 with data from 2001 to 2003 indicated that the prevalence of psychiatric disorders did not change over the decade of the 1990s (about 30% of the population had a diagnosable disorder). In other words, the disorders did not appear to be getting more common over the ten-year time frame. Furthermore, the percent of individuals being treated for psychiatric disorders increased. At first glance, this would seem to be really good news. Unfortunately, only about half of those treated for a psychiatric disorder actually had a psychiatric disorder; many were apparently treated for nonspecific symptoms but not a disorder. The great majority of patients with psychiatric disorders got *no* treatment. Adding to this depressing news was the fact that major disparities in treatment continued to exist and were associated with race and social status; being poor and in a minority population typically meant limited or no psychiatric care.

The findings of the NCS-R caused us to do some quick calculations based on our understanding of the psychiatric literature. We were interested in estimating how many patients with a treatable disorder like major depression are effectively treated in our current US health care delivery system. Sadly, we think it is very few—maybe 10 successes at most out of every 100 individuals with depression. Why is this the case? First, even when individuals with depression go to their doctor (almost always a nonpsychiatrist), they only have about a one in two chance of being recognized as being depressed. Of the 50% who are recognized as being depressed, about half get the wrong treatment (e.g., they get something for sleep or anxiety but not for depression). Those who do get an antidepressant medication may also not fare well: Some do not take their medication as prescribed (called "poor compliance" by doctors), and others experience side effects that limit their ability to take the medication (e.g., sexual dysfunction or nausea). Finally, the current drugs are not 100% effective. Thus, we estimate that only about 10 in 100 are effectively treated for their depression. This is a rather pathetic performance for a country that prides itself on its health care and spends so much of its gross national product on health care costs.

The point of this discussion is that psychiatric disorders are significant problems for human beings and societies. They also appear to be under-recognized and undertreated. Subsequent chapters in this book will explore these topics in greater detail in an attempt to foster a broader understanding both of psychiatry as a field and of the nature of mental disorders. We will consider what psychiatrists actually do, what illnesses they diagnose, how they treat these disorders, and how they function within the health care delivery system. Along the way we will also consider factors that make psychiatric disorders so common and describe what is known and not known about the causes of psychiatric disorders from genetic and neuroscience perspectives. We will end with some cautionary notes for patients and families and with some thoughts about current trends in the field and its future direction. Based on developments across multiple areas, we believe the field of psychiatry is well positioned for major advances over the next several decades and certainly over the 21st century. These advances will affect how individuals with psychiatric disorders are diagnosed and treated and will therefore influence their overall outcome and quality of life.

Take-Home Messages

- Psychiatric disorders are common. Indeed, it is highly likely that all the readers of this book have personal experience with psychiatric dysfunction in themselves, their family, or their friends.
  The disorders are just too common for this not to be the case.

- Psychiatric disorders are real problems, as defined by the suffering, disability, and death that they cause. For these reasons, these disorders fall under the realm of medicine and the care of doctors of medicine.

- Psychiatrists are medical doctors who specialize in the treatment of mental disorders. Because of their training, psychiatrists have the greatest expertise regarding the diagnosis of and the range of available treatments for psychiatric illness.

- Finally, psychiatric disorders are widely misunderstood.
  The remainder of this book is aimed at helping to diminish these misperceptions and the stigma associated with the disorders and their treatment.

··· *two* ···

What Illnesses Do Psychiatrists Treat?

Psychiatric disorders reflect dysfunction of the human mind and behavior and are diagnosed according to specific criteria. As noted in Chapter 1, dysfunction of the human mind results in symptoms in three primary spheres: thinking (cognition), emotion (meaning), and motivation (ability to set and achieve goals). These disorders can also produce a variety of physical (or "neurovegetative") symptoms that include changes in appetite, sleep, sexual function, and energy level, among others. Some people develop symptoms suggestive of other medical or neurological disorders, such as heart palpitations, shortness of breath, pain, and memory disturbances. Additionally, patients with serious medical and neurological disorders can develop psychiatric disorders (e.g., people with diabetes are prone to develop depression), with adverse effects likely affecting the outcome of both conditions.

All medical disorders, psychiatric and otherwise, are diagnosed based on signs and symptoms that are characteristic of a given disorder. "Symptoms" are complaints that patients bring to the attention of their doctor, while "signs" are features of a disorder that the physician observes during examination. But a major difference between psychiatric disorders and other medical disorders concerns the usefulness of laboratory tests for diagnosis. Currently, psychiatric diagnosis largely relies upon historical information that patients, as well as their families and friends, provide. Unlike illnesses that internists treat, for which results from blood tests, x-rays, electrocardiograms, and blood pressure monitoring are extremely useful diagnostically, primary psychiatric disorders cannot be diagnosed from laboratory tests; indeed, there are presently *no* laboratory studies that reliably establish their diagnosis.

That said, laboratory tests and physical examination are useful to psychiatrists in determining whether other medical or neurological disorders are contributing to a patient's symptoms. Such approaches are valuable for overall management, but they do not help in distinguishing one psychiatric disorder from another or even in determining whether a psychiatric disorder is present. For instance, a psychiatrist is likely to order blood tests to check for thyroid dysfunction in a patient with anxiety. If thyroid function is abnormal, correcting the thyroid problem is likely to reduce the patient's symptoms of anxiety. However, there are no laboratory findings that are uniquely abnormal in primary anxiety disorders, such as panic disorder or generalized anxiety disorder. We would note that blood or urine testing for alcohol and abused drugs can provide important information when evaluating and monitoring psychiatric and medical symptoms. Thus, this type of testing is routinely used by psychiatrists when they suspect that drug abuse is contributing to a patient's problems.

We should mention that genetic testing will likely provide clinically useful psychiatric diagnostic information in the future. But as of 2009, we do not believe that such testing is useful in helping psychiatrists to diagnose any primary psychiatric disorder. A neuropsychiatric disorder called Huntington's disease is an exception to this statement. This illness runs in families such that about half of each generation will inherit the illness from an affected parent. Geneticists refer to this pattern of inheritance as "autosomal dominant," meaning that if you get the abnormal gene, you get the illness. Neurologists treat persons with Huntington's disease more often than do psychiatrists since the illness involves neurological symptoms, including characteristic jerky movements (called "chorea") together with deteriorating memory and thinking abilities. However, sometimes the first symptoms of Huntington's disease are changes in personality or the development of a significant depression. Since depression can occur for many reasons, genetic testing in individuals at familial risk can help determine whether they carry the gene for Huntington's disease and thus whether their depression might be an initial symptom. Otherwise, apart from a few exceptions like this, we believe that the use of genetic testing to identify primary psychiatric disorders, given the current state of knowledge, is very premature and likely to be more harmful to patients than helpful. We would in any case advise people not to send genetic material to laboratories for testing pertaining to any illness without the guidance of knowledgeable physicians and genetic counselors. Advances in genetics are very important in psychiatry, but at this time, genetic testing is a research, not clinical, tool.

The current system used for psychiatric diagnosis in the United States is called "DSM-Four" (DSM-IV: *Diagnostic and Statistical Manual of Mental*

Disorders, Fourth Edition, published by the American Psychiatric Association in 1994). DSM-IV, and its predecessor DSM-III (1980), grew out of efforts to develop a more reliable system for categorizing mental disorders than had existed in the first two editions of the manual. As noted in Chapter 1, most psychiatric disorders can now be diagnosed very reliably, meaning that there is excellent agreement among psychiatrists about the signs and symptoms that define a disorder and that the signs and symptoms exhibited by a patient remain consistent during repeated examinations of the patient. The validity of psychiatric diagnoses has proven more difficult, given that the underlying brain dysfunction that leads to psychiatric illness is not well understood. Thus, validation of psychiatric disorders does not presently rely on neuropathology (changes in the anatomy and structure of the brain) or on altered brain chemistry. Rather, it is anchored in four primary criteria: (1) good clinical description based on specific diagnostic criteria; (2) the ability to separate one disorder from another disorder; (3) a family history indicating that the disorder runs in families; and (4) a characteristic pattern of symptoms that can be recognized over the long-term course of the disorder. Until researchers discover the underlying brain abnormalities that cause specific psychiatric disorders, validity will likely continue to be defined by these criteria. Such illnesses as major depression, bipolar disorder, schizophrenia, and alcoholism are well validated using these criteria and are thus among the most useful psychiatric diagnoses. Other diagnoses, such as multiple personality disorder (dissociative identity disorder), conversion disorder (characterized by symptoms such as pseudo-seizures and pseudoparalysis that mimic neurological dysfunction), and even some types of post-traumatic stress disorder, are much less well validated, meaning that their utility for describing a patient's course of illness is much more limited.

When assessing behavior that indicates the possibility of a psychiatric disorder, clinicians must also consider the individual's social and cultural circumstances. Beliefs that are considered acceptable within one culture may be considered abnormal in another culture. Furthermore, behaviors that are acceptable in one social group may be completely forbidden in another. For these reasons, psychiatrists often talk with a patient's social circle of family and friends in order to understand whether they view the patient's symptoms as abnormal. For example, many people don't believe in faith healing or "speaking in tongues." Nonetheless, there are religions and cultures that do. Thus, when a person has started "speaking in tongues," it is important to know whether others in the same culture see the symptom or behavior as abnormal. The ability to evaluate and treat mental disorders in a culturally sensitive manner that takes ethnic and religious differences into account can be a significant challenge for psychiatrists and other mental health professionals.

A detailed discussion about the signs and symptoms of various psychiatric disorders is beyond the scope of this chapter. Rather, we have three goals: (1) to present an overview of the major categories of mental disorders that general psychiatrists encounter in adults and older adolescents; (2) to discuss how these common conditions are diagnosed and treated; and (3) to demonstrate that the same group of psychiatric illnesses, such as depressive disorders, can have many faces. For more complete descriptions of psychiatric disorders, readers should consult DSM-IV or leading textbooks of psychiatry, some of which are listed in the bibliography at the end of this book.

A Few Definitions

As is true of all of medicine, psychiatry is in some ways a language unto itself. It is said that Hawaiians have about 100 words to describe ocean waves and Alaskans have a similar number to describe snow. Similarly, psychiatrists have a large number of words to describe human emotions and thinking. In this section, we will highlight a few of these terms to set the stage for later discussion of several specific types of mental disorders. The terms we have chosen to highlight are among the ones most commonly used and are thus most likely to be encountered regularly by patients and their families.

The term *psychosis* (or the adjective *psychotic*) is very important in psychiatry. It refers both to patterns of thinking and behavior and to a class of disorders. Perhaps the simplest and most useful definition of psychosis is the presence of delusions, hallucinations, and/or markedly disorganized speech or behavior. In politically incorrect but popular nonpsychiatric jargon, these symptoms are what most people mean when they describe someone as "insane" or "crazy." The term *delusion* refers to a fixed false belief that is out of context in the patient's culture. Examples include the belief that you are getting special messages from space aliens who are controlling your thinking, or the belief that the President of the United States is madly in love with you (unless of course you are the President's spouse). Another common psychotic symptom is called a *delusion of reference*. Here patients interpret the actions or comments of others (including on television and radio) as being directed specifically toward themselves and having special meaning for them. Such referential thinking might be manifest by such comments as "The man on TV is talking about the bad things I have done." Patients rigidly hold to delusional beliefs even in the face of contrary evidence, and it is their unwavering adherence to such beliefs that may be the most defining characteristic of delusions.

Hallucinations, on the other hand, are false sensory perceptions, usually involving hearing voices of people who aren't present (auditory hallucinations) or seeing things that aren't present (visual hallucinations). Often hallucinations reflect some of the delusional ideas that a patient has (e.g., hearing the voices of the space aliens who are controlling your thinking). Other hallucinations can involve false smells (olfactory hallucinations) or feelings of being physically touched or manipulated (somatic hallucinations). In short, hallucinations can occur in any of our senses. Psychotic disorganized speech can range from markedly illogical statements to "tangentiality" (marked digression in response to a question to the point that the question is not really answered) or "incoherence" (inability to put thoughts into words at the level of individual sentences; sometimes called "word salad"). Psychiatrists refer to patterns of disorganized speech as a *formal thought disorder*, meaning a defect in the *form* that thought takes when it is put into words. This is different from a defect in the *content* of thought (like a delusion). In interpreting psychotic symptoms and signs, context is everything. For example, some politicians are masters at being "tangential" in their responses; that is, they never really answer the question being asked but tell you what they want you to hear. It is the overall context of the thought disorder that helps psychiatrists to recognize it as "psychotic."

The term *obsession* (or *obsessive*) is commonly used and is often misunderstood by patients. For psychiatrists, an obsession is a persistent thought, idea, or impulse that is experienced as intrusive, unwanted, and anxiety-provoking. Patients generally struggle against these kinds of thoughts and recognize them as inappropriate (as opposed to a delusion, which is believed strongly and rigidly). Examples include intrusive thoughts about germs or illness. Often obsessions are accompanied by *compulsions*, actions and rituals that are done to diminish the anxiety that the obsession produces. Examples include repeatedly checking the stove to make sure it is turned off or repeated bouts of hand washing or showering because of fear of germs. Importantly, afflicted persons recognize these obsessions and compulsions to be abnormal, but they can't get the idea out of their head and can't stop doing the activity without marked anxiety. A French term for obsessive-compulsive disorder referred to it as the "doubting disease," a fairly accurate descriptor of the angst that these symptoms cause: No matter how many times something is checked, no matter how many times one showers, there remains doubt that things are not quite correct and must be done again. In older terms, obsessive-compulsive symptoms fell into the category of "neurotic" behaviors. The term *neurotic* is not commonly used in psychiatry these days, and it has a vague definition that largely conveys the idea that these types of symptoms and disorders cause anxiety and dysfunction but are not psychotic. A common adage used to distinguish neurosis from psychosis states that "neurotics build castles in the air, while psychotics live in them."

Anthropologists suggest that humans have six primary emotions (happiness, sadness, fear, anger, surprise, and disgust; some add a seventh, contempt). These states reflect similar feelings across cultures and are associated with similar facial expressions in human populations throughout the world. Defects in emotion are very common in psychiatric disorders, and psychiatrists have numerous terms to describe emotional states. For psychiatrists, the term *mood* refers to a sustained emotional state that colors a person's perception of the world. Terms like *sad*, *anxious*, *euphoric*, and *irritable* are among those used to describe mood. The term *affect* refers to observable behaviors that reflect the underlying mood state. Affect may be described with terms like *blunted*, *labile*, and *inappropriate*. In some ways, mood is like the climate of a region, reflecting a longer-term pattern, while affect describes the current weather. Some psychiatrists vary from these definitions and use *mood* to describe what patients say about how they feel and *affect* to describe what they observe in talking with patients. Both definitions are acceptable, but it is useful to know which one is being used when the terms are discussed.

Two other terms that are frequently used by psychiatrists are *insight* and *judgment*. Insight refers to whether patients understand that they have an illness, that the illness has symptoms and consequences, and that they should seek help. Judgment, on the other hand, refers to whether patients have the ability to understand the norms of society and to adjust their behaviors to meet those norms. Defects in insight and judgment are major problems associated with some psychiatric disorders and are responsible for many patients failing to seek care or to follow through with care. In addition, defects in these areas may lead patients to exhibit inappropriate behaviors in public or social settings.

Mood Disorders

Patients suffering from mood disorders make up the great bulk of many psychiatric practices. This fact reflects how common mood disorders are in the general population. Mood disorders represent major problems with emotions as demonstrated by persistent sadness (major depression), elation (mania), and/or irritability. Importantly, changes in mood alone are not sufficient to diagnose these disorders. They are also associated with bodily changes and defects in cognition and motivation. For example, patients with "major depression" exhibit persistent problems in the majority of nine different categories of symptoms. These nine symptom categories include problems with mood (feeling down or sad), appetite (weight loss or gain), sleep (insomnia, hypersomnia, or early morning awakening), energy (fatigue), loss of interest in pleasurable activities (e.g., sex or hobbies), concentration (inability to focus thoughts), self-esteem, physical movement (nervous pacing or hand wringing called "psychomotor agitation" or markedly decreased movement called "psychomotor retardation"), and thoughts about death (suicidal thoughts or suicidal plans). It is important to note that everyone feels sad at some point(s) in his or her life. The disorder called depression is much more than just sadness and reflects a symptom constellation that can persist for months or years.

Although the term *major depression* suggests a single disorder, there are in fact many types. In some people, symptoms develop over a few days and seem to come out of the blue. Afflicted persons may be otherwise healthy but show a dramatic change in behavior. They may become unable to function and may stay in bed all day. Their mood may become sullen and withdrawn. Their motivation declines, their thinking slows, and their ability to focus attention becomes incapacitated. Making even a simple decision becomes like an act of Congress for them. They are unable to experience pleasure ("anhedonia"). Sometimes, these symptoms are much worse in the morning but get better as the day progresses ("diurnal variation"). Depression with these kinds of symptoms has sometimes been called "melancholic depression," and those afflicted with it can also develop psychotic symptoms. They may hear voices telling them that they are evil and worthless. They may believe that they are the cause of the evils of the world or that they deserve punishment for past "sins." This type of depression is referred to as "major depression with psychosis." It is important to distinguish psychotic from nonpsychotic depression because the treatment approaches for each are quite different. For example, the person with psychotic depression generally does not respond well to antidepressant medication unless it is coupled with antipsychotic medication. The treatment of nonpsychotic depression does not require the use of antipsychotic medication. Also, treatment approaches using talk therapy (psychotherapy) may differ if psychotic symptoms are present.

If a person with depression develops a manic episode, yet another treatment approach is required. A manic episode is defined by the development of several of the following symptoms. The individual feels really good, in fact way too good (euphoric), and this feeling may evolve into irritable and agitated behavior. This euphoric mood may be accompanied by an overestimated sense of self (grandiose to the point of believing that one has special powers or is actually a chosen person) and less need for sleep such that the person wakes up super-charged after only a few hours of sleep. People exhibiting manic symptoms often have a formal thought disorder, and their speech is excessive, rapid, and often uninterruptable. They also have trouble paying attention, their minds jump rapidly from topic to topic, and their thoughts may be hard to follow. Psychiatrists sometimes refer to the rapid digressive speech seen during mania as "flight of ideas," a useful descriptor that captures the quickly changing content of thought. Behavior becomes inappropriate and may involve risky sexual behaviors, spending sprees, gambling, and excessive drug use. Such manic episodes are often distinct from major depressive episodes; however, sometimes a person can alternate between manic and depressive episodes over very short intervals. At times, it may even appear that a person is having a mixed episode with symptoms of both mania and depression. When a person is in a depressive episode but has a history of previous manic episodes, the appropriate psychiatric diagnosis is "bipolar disorder" (formerly "manic-depressive illness"), and the treatment of the current depressive episode is once again different from the two other types of depression discussed previously. In this example, a type of medicine called a "mood stabilizer" is necessary. Counseling is also warranted, although it would likely focus on different issues than those presented by a person without a history of a manic episode. From a diagnostic standpoint, the presence of even one full-blown episode of mania is sufficient to qualify for the diagnosis of bipolar disorder. Some individuals with this disorder have recurrent bouts of mania but not depression.

Another type of depression is exemplified by people who become addicted to drugs of abuse and develop depressive symptoms. A dose of cocaine, for example, may help them feel better temporarily, but whenever they are away from cocaine, they may become acutely and severely depressed and have strong thoughts of suicide. This type of depression is time-linked to the use and withdrawal of the drug. The initial treatment strategy is likely to be different from the approaches used for the other types of depressions previously discussed. Sometimes, these depressions go away if the person stays away from cocaine for several days. But even if the depression gets better, the drug addiction requires aggressive treatment in order to help the person begin the long process of recovery. The depression may get better after a week, but the irresistible desire to resume using cocaine drives this person's behavior. Treatment approaches usually require a combination of psychosocial support (frequently with 12-step programs), medications (sometimes), and an emphasis on encouraging the person to work on building a meaningful life away from drugs.

Many older persons develop depressions that are time-linked to other chronic medical illnesses such as heart disease or diabetes. Such depressions may be long-lasting, and the symptoms, although present and disabling, are sometimes subtle. The depression makes the heart disease worse, and the heart disease makes the depression worse. Treatments for these types of depression often involve the coordinated effort of a psychiatrist and an internist or cardiologist in order to address both the mood disorder and the medical disorder. Treating one disorder but not the other is not likely to be as beneficial as treating both. Treatment involves medicines to treat the depression, medicines to treat the heart disease, counseling, and, very importantly, a major emphasis on lifestyle changes, including increased exercise and improved diet. Since many older patients with heart disease and diabetes are on a large number of medications, the medical training of a psychiatrist becomes essential for evaluating the risks and the benefits of adding antidepressant medications and for anticipating the potential for drug interactions. Many other medical conditions, not all of them chronic, are associated with depression. Some examples include depression following the birth of a child or following a significant injury. In all of these conditions, optimal care requires coordination among a diverse group of health care providers.

Another form of depressive disorder is one manifested by some people who have persistent but somewhat milder mood dysfunction. These persistent depressive symptoms cause long-lasting distress but don't meet criteria for a diagnosis of major depression. This type of depression is called "dysthymic disorder," whose long-standing baseline depressive symptoms can be punctuated by periods of full-blown major depression. Similarly, some patients with manic symptoms have forms of the disorder that don't meet criteria for bipolar disorder and may be diagnosed with "bipolar II disorder" or "cyclothymia." These lower-level mood disorders are much less well validated than major depression and bipolar disorder (type I). Thus, how useful they are as descriptors is a debate in the field.

Why do people get mood disorders? What parts of the brain malfunction in the various types of mood disorders? In what way are life events involved in the development of mood disorders? How are such environmental factors as diet, activity level, and obesity involved? Are such early life stressors as abuse and neglect capable of influencing brain development in a manner that predisposes a person to depression later in life? Various depressive disorders are known to be strongly influenced by genes. How are our genes involved? How do genes and environment interact to set the stage for these various disorders? These are but a few of the fascinating questions that are being addressed by current psychiatric research. We don't have complete answers today, but our knowledge of the causes of these disorders will no doubt increase with advancing science.

Anxiety Disorders

Animals, including humans, are programmed to respond to certain situations with fear. Separating young animals from their nurturing parent leads to fearful and panicked responses. Similarly, exposing animals to natural predators can trigger a major fear response. The particular brain systems that are involved in fear responses are becoming better defined. Given the importance of fear as a primary human emotion, it is no surprise that there is a group of psychiatric disorders defined by a dysregulation of fear responses. Symptoms may show up as sudden waves of panic or as a more pervasive generalized anxiety. Some of the brain systems involved with fear overlap with brain systems involved with depression. Therefore, it is common for anxiety to accompany various depressive disorders. On the other hand, there are certain anxiety disorders that can occur in the absence of depression.

The anxiety disorder that may have the most overt and dramatic presentation is panic disorder, which is defined by frequent panic attacks, concerns about future attacks, and often changes in behavior to diminish the risk of an attack. What is a panic attack? In the classic presentation, people have a sudden onset of intense fear that they are dying or having a heart attack. It's almost as if a fear alarm has gone off by accident. They become very afraid, breathe rapidly (hyperventilate), and often experience chest pain and abnormal heartbeats. Numbness and tingling in the hands and feet can also be experienced and often are the result of hyperventilation. Symptoms may last for several minutes and then subside. A panic attack is a frightening event and often leads a person to seek treatment in an emergency room or a doctor's office.

Why people experience occasional panic attacks isn't known. Why some people develop these attacks on a regular basis is also not known. What is known is that humans are very good at associating symptoms with other events that occur at the same time; this is actually one of the ways that we learn new things. It is not uncommon for a person to associate panic attacks with being in a certain environment such as a crowded place. When such an association occurs, a person is likely to become fearful of being in certain places and to start avoiding them. This is called "panic disorder with agoraphobia" (a term that generally means "fear of open spaces;" actually "fear of the market place" [agora] in Greek). Fortunately, many medications and various psychotherapies can be very effective at helping patients who suffer from panic disorder and its consequences.

Humans are social animals. Yet there are many people who develop a condition known as "social phobia" ("social anxiety disorder"). This disorder is characterized by a marked, excessive fear of social situations that most people would find comfortable or at least tolerable. More than mild shyness, the disorder can lead to marked avoidance of those situations that make the person nervous and can severely interfere with his or her everyday life. When does shyness evolve into social phobia? Why are some individuals very much "people persons," while others are slightly uncomfortable in social situations and still others are incapacitated by such interactions? What part of our brain is responsible for these variations? What kinds of interactions of genes and environment predispose to this type of anxiety? Again, questions abound, but we don't have great answers . . . yet. We do know, however, that social phobia is another disorder involving fear that can be quite responsive to various interventions.

Another type of anxiety disorder can occur in response to experiencing an extraordinarily intimidating or frightening event. Some people exposed to such disturbing events develop post-traumatic stress disorder (PTSD), which can lead to substantial changes in the ability to function. They may re-experience the event via thoughts or dreams, avoid situations or thoughts that evoke reminders of the event, and show enhanced arousal (e.g., sleeping difficulty, increased fear responses to various stimuli, and increased alertness to certain situations). These symptoms can become persistent. Based on studies involving individuals who survived terrorist attacks in Oklahoma City and New York City, it appears that many people show at least some signs of distress and features of PTSD following major adverse events. Our combat troops are clearly exposed to life-threatening and gruesome events, and it is not surprising that many develop PTSD. Individuals who develop early, dramatic symptoms of emotional numbness to events and people around them and avoidance of interpersonal interactions and obligations are at highest risk for persistent PTSD. So are persons with preexisting psychiatric disorders (e.g., depression or personality disorders) prior to the traumatic event. But contrary to popular belief, most people do not go on to have full-blown PTSD. It appears that many people can tolerate exposure to intimidating and frightening events without developing chronic symptoms of PTSD, whereas others are quite susceptible. Why are some people much more susceptible to PTSD than others? What fear systems in the brain are involved in this anxiety disorder, and do these systems overlap with the other anxiety disorders that we have discussed?

Several other disorders involve symptoms of anxiety. People may experience short periods of acute anxiety that are triggered by life events. Some people develop specific phobias, such as a fear of flying. Many people are generally nervous by nature and are chronically worried. Such people can't control their worries, and their anxiety is associated with sleep problems, difficulties with concentration, and irritability, which can significantly interfere with everyday function. This latter disorder is known as "generalized anxiety disorder." Again, if recognized, these forms of anxiety can usually be successfully treated.

Finally, obsessive-compulsive disorder (OCD) is also included among the illnesses classified as anxiety disorders. OCD is characterized by persistent obsessions, that is, recurrent thoughts that become very intrusive. Even though people with OCD recognize such thoughts as being abnormal, unproductive, and interfering, they can't get rid of them. Sometimes these thoughts lead to compulsive, repetitive actions, such as repeated hand washing, checking behaviors, hoarding, or counting behaviors, which can be extraordinarily disruptive. Some forms of OCD are fairly mild and respond well to treatment. Less common, more severe forms can be very hard to treat and can ruin lives. The brain circuitry involved in these disorders overlaps somewhat with the depression circuitry in the brain, and these two disorders can coexist. In OCD, it is almost as if the brain's circuitry gets stuck in a repetitive cycle and can't reset itself. The more we learn about the anatomy and chemistry of these circuits, the more likely we will be able to develop better treatments.

Psychotic Disorders

As explained earlier, psychotic symptoms include hallucinations, delusions, bizarre behavior, and formal thought disorder. There are primary illnesses in which these symptoms are prominent, and there are other disorders in which these symptoms, although perhaps not central to the illness, are often present. For instance, in Alzheimer's disease, the key symptom is loss of memory. But as the disease progresses, the majority of patients develop hallucinations and/ or delusions, and it may account for more psychotic symptoms in the elderly than any other disorder. Similarly, delirium is a disorder that results in fairly abrupt changes in orientation (awareness of one's surroundings), attention, and concentration. It can also be associated with psychotic symptoms, such as hallucinations and delusions. The subtype of depression associated with psychotic symptoms that we mentioned previously would also be considered a psychotic disorder. So would bipolar disorder if the patient hears voices or believes he is God. Thus, some patients with bipolar disorder have a psychotic illness.

There is one disorder (or more likely a group of disorders), however, in which psychotic symptoms are the central feature of the illness. That disorder is schizophrenia. Its core features include a combination of hallucinations, delusions, and formal thought disorder (i.e., disorganized speech). Along with these active and often dramatic "positive symptoms" comes a hollowing out of the person's personality that results in what are called "negative symptoms." By this we mean that people with schizophrenia become more isolated, unmotivated, and withdrawn. They don't enjoy things and may be unable to interact comfortably with others. Certain cognitive abilities (i.e., memory and reasoning) also change with this disorder, and difficulties in thinking clearly and coherently may be the most disabling aspects of the disorder. Imagine that you hear voices that you are convinced are real, yet you can't see anyone. Imagine that you believe that people are spying on you or are trying to poison you. Try to imagine this in the context of your brain being less able to understand routine information in an efficient manner. Your brain may not even allow you to express your thoughts in a coherent enough manner to be understood by those who want to help you. You may find that cigarettes (or, more accurately, the nicotine in cigarettes) help you think a bit better, and so you smoke. You may find that certain drugs of abuse help you escape a bit, and so you start to use illegal substances and get hooked on them.

As you can imagine, schizophrenia is a horrible illness. It tends to be a chronic, life-long problem. There are effective drug treatments (i.e., antipsychotic medications) that can help quiet the positive symptoms, but they probably do little for the negative symptoms and the cognitive impairment. Nonthreatening psychological support can be of great help. Clubhouse settings where people with this illness can learn how to perform certain tasks that will enable them to hold down a job and feel better about themselves can be lifesaving.

What goes wrong in the brains of individuals with schizophrenia? We are learning a lot about changes that may occur in the brain during early childhood development. Interestingly, even though such changes may be present very early in life, they usually don't lead to severe symptoms until adolescence or even later. We are also learning about various genetic factors that increase the risk for these illnesses and about various environmental changes that may interact with such genes. Current and future research discoveries should give us a greater opportunity to develop even better treatments for this illness than we have now.

A fairly common disorder that probably represents a poorly understood interface between bipolar disorder and schizophrenia is schizoaffective disorder. Individuals with this disorder have prominent periods of mood dysregulation (mania and/or depression) and long-lasting psychotic symptoms that persist during periods in which mood symptoms improve. The mechanisms causing schizoaffective disorder, like those for schizophrenia and bipolar disorder, are not well understood, but likely reflect complex interactions among the brain circuits that underlie mood, thinking, and motivation. Treatment of this complex disorder is difficult and requires a combination of the approaches outlined previously for schizophrenia and bipolar disorder.

Finally, psychiatrists also encounter patients suffering from an entity called "delusional disorder." Individuals with this disorder have chronic and fixed false beliefs (usually delusions of a persecutory or referential nature), but they don't have mood symptoms or the hallucinations, disorganized thinking, and bizarre behavior of other psychotic disorders. These individuals often go untreated for long periods of time unless they become agitated by their symptoms or they start to cause problems for their families and friends. Treatment is typically with antipsychotic medications, but the chronic symptoms can be difficult to control.

Drug Use Disorders

Through evolution, humans have inherited several elementary brain systems that are crucial for our survival. Some of these systems generate an instinctive need to reproduce and govern our emotions. Others promote the impulse to nurture and protect our young. Jaak Panksepp, a leader in evolutionary neurobiology, describes seven such brain systems, including one called "seeking." This system is responsible for many appetitive behaviors (e.g., seeking food and sex) and may be the core of what we call "motivation." Animals have a drive to seek out and explore. This drive can be pleasurable and self-reinforcing, and it is likely to be one of the major brain systems hijacked by drugs of abuse. Abused drugs substitute for or enhance the activity of normal brain chemicals that are responsible for the normal and healthy regulation of such brain systems. Such drugs initially feel really good. They literally turn on our internal pleasure systems and are rewarding. The problem is that repeated drug use begins to change the system, and the brain begins to need the external substance just to feel normal.

Drug use disorders range from acute intoxication with a substance to frequent use that gets a person into trouble (drug abuse) to such chronic use that the brain actually changes and a person can't function without the drug. In the latter case, the person's life becomes dominated by the need for the drug. Without it, the individual has dramatic and potentially fatal withdrawal reactions (drug dependence). The brain has become so dependent on the drug that when the drug is absent for an extended period of time, the brain tries to compensate and inadvertently causes the body to go through painful and possibly lethal adjustments. These withdrawal reactions differ depending on the nature of the drug; that is, they are dependent on how the drug chemically resets certain parts of the brain's seeking and reward systems.

When we think of drugs of abuse, we naturally think of illegal substances such as heroin, cocaine, methamphetamine, PCP (phencyclidine), and marijuana. All of these drugs influence parts of the brain's central reward system in different ways. Thus, they have different pleasurable effects and, eventually, different devastating effects. However, the two drugs that plague our society financially and medically more than any other are two common legal drugs—tobacco (nicotine) and alcohol. By far, tobacco and alcohol account for more costs to the US economy in terms of health costs, lost productivity, and disability than all of the other abused drugs combined. Despite this, we, as a society, tend to become outraged about the use of illegal substances, but perhaps are less perturbed by the use of these more devastating "legal" agents. This is not to say that the other drugs would not become greater problems if they were more readily available and more socially acceptable.

Cigarettes are best thought of as a drug delivery system that transports nicotine very effectively to the brain. Anyone in the 30 to 40% of the population that is or has been addicted to cigarettes can testify how hard it is to kick this habit. The medical consequences of smoking are more costly and more lethal than any other drug, including alcohol. There is nothing healthy about cigarettes. A little bit of smoking is bad for you, and a lot of smoking is much worse.

Alcohol is the second most costly drug of abuse. Here the story is much more complicated, however. Many people drink in moderation, and there are certain physical and social benefits from occasional drinking. The problem with alcohol is that a significant minority of people becomes dependent on this drug. Their lives become dominated by alcohol, leading to dramatic social and physical consequences. The social consequences can kill the drinker as well as others through, for example, drunk driving and violence. If a person dependent on alcohol decides to stop suddenly and without assistance, he or she may experience a dramatic and potentially lethal withdrawal syndrome that can range in intensity. The most severe form of alcohol withdrawal is called "delirium tremens" ("DTs"). When this type of withdrawal occurs, it is a medical emergency. As its name implies, DTs cause delirium—that is, confusion and agitation plus tremors ("shakes"). Dysregulation of blood pressure and heart rate is common. Various organ systems may stop working correctly, and if blood pressure or cardiac or respiratory systems become too dysregulated, death can occur. Most people who abuse alcohol don't experience DTs upon withdrawal, but have milder forms of withdrawal, including early-morning awakening and tremulousness ("morning shakes"). A hallmark of alcoholism is drinking in the morning (or just after arising from sleep).

The reason for this urge, just as for the first morning cigarette, is to "treat" early symptoms of withdrawal. Importantly, alcohol and nicotine are very effective in treating their own withdrawal symptoms. This sets up a horribly vicious cycle where the need to drink or smoke may largely result from self-treatment of withdrawal. Some alcoholics also experience generalized seizures as part of their withdrawal syndrome, and thus, alcoholism is among the considerations when doctors evaluate patients who have new onset of seizures.

The specific syndromes of intoxication or withdrawal associated with each category of drug are fascinating from a scientific perspective and devastating from an individual perspective. One of the most frequent reasons patients come to the attention of psychiatrists in the emergency room setting is the involvement of drugs of abuse in the patients' behavior. Such patients may be experiencing suicidal thoughts while coming down from a cocaine high. They may be violent and agitated from "angel dust" (PCP, phencyclidine) or methamphetamine. They may be brought in by the police for inappropriate behavior while intoxicated with alcohol. In persons with primary psychiatric disorders, the mixture of the acute and chronic effects of drugs of abuse can lead to behaviors that require aggressive psychiatric treatment.

The effects of such drugs of abuse on the brain remain long after the drugs are discontinued. Persons kicking a drug or alcohol habit have a life-long challenge ahead of them. In order for the brain to reset, a person needs to be abstinent for an extended period of time, months and perhaps years. This usually requires tremendous support from many sources in order to prevent the patient's relapse. Experts in the field of recovery from substance disorders believe that long-term success at remaining abstinent often requires that recovering addicts develop a new life philosophy that includes improving their self-esteem and the ways in which they interact with others. Humans are amazing in their capacity to help themselves beat addictions by modifying behaviors that require the highest levels of conscious and adaptive thinking.

Cognitive Disorders

Why discuss cognitive disorders like Alzheimer's disease (dementia of the Alzheimer type, DAT) in a book about psychiatry? We've already touched on one reason: the fact that DAT often presents psychotic symptoms as the disease progresses. Another reason is historical: DAT was first described by Alois Alzheimer in 1906, and the disease was named after him in 1910 by Emil Kraepelin; both Alzheimer and Kraepelin were psychiatrists. But DAT is actually a disorder whose treatment falls into several domains—psychiatry, neurology, internal medicine, and geriatrics, with general physicians often involved in the initial diagnosis and long-term management of persons with this disorder.

DAT is characterized by progressive deterioration in multiple brain functions. Memory deterioration is clearly involved and is a hallmark of the disorder. Also, changes occur in organizational and planning skills, orientation skills, and math and verbal skills. In other words, defects occur in many if not all higher intellectual functions. In addition, persons with this disorder develop many behavioral (noncognitive) symptoms. Personality changes are frequent and can include suspiciousness, irritability, or inappropriateness in conversations. Depression is also common. Hallucinations and delusions may occur as the illness becomes more severe. Unfortunately, some people also become so severely agitated, irritable, and combative that their families are unable to care for them at home. At that point, such patients need inpatient care and often require the expertise of an inpatient geriatric psychiatry unit.

The onset of DAT is subtle and gradual. Once it starts, it invariably progresses, although in its very mild stages, it may be many years before the disorder has substantial impact on a person's activities. Eventually, a person will be unable to accomplish complex tasks of daily living such as managing finances or driving a car. The ability to recognize family members becomes impaired. The patient's suspicion regarding the intent of loved ones is an especially difficult symptom for family members to understand and can lead to marital and familial stress. Agitation or loss of bowel and bladder control may be events that make it difficult for family members to manage the individual, and nursing home placement becomes an unfortunate, but necessary, alternative. The important point is that all of these symptoms reflect degeneration of multiple brain systems. While families sometimes think that patients are "making things up," the symptoms result from a failing brain and are very real.

There are drug treatments that can help slow the progression of the disorder . . . somewhat. Currently, such treatments, although useful, are very small steps in the right direction. Psychological support of patients and their families is also extremely helpful. Group support provided by the expertise of the Alzheimer's Association is highly recommended and can be a godsend for families, particularly for the individuals most directly involved in providing day-to-day care for the patient.

Progress in understanding DAT is dramatic and exciting, and research has benefited from the perspectives of many fields. We are close to being able to use brain imaging methods to identify the illness in people years before symptoms are evident. One pathological finding, and a hallmark of DAT, is the abnormal accumulation in the brain of a chemical called beta-amyloid.

It is likely that this amyloid accumulation plays an important, if not major, role in causing the symptoms of the illness. Treatments are being developed that may be able to alter the accumulation of amyloid. Therefore, it is possible that in the future we will be able to diagnose brain changes that cause the illness years before symptoms begin and then to start a person on treatment to delay substantially, or perhaps even prevent, the onset of the illness. These possibilities were considered science fiction in the mid-1990s. Now they are realistic goals.

There are several other illnesses that lead to a deterioration in memory and thinking as well as major behavioral changes. After DAT, the second most common dementia related to degeneration of the brain is called "dementia with Lewy bodies" (DLB), its name referring to the accumulation of abnormal substances, so-called Lewy bodies, found in the brains of patients with this disease. Scientists are just beginning to understand the nature of these abnormal substances and the cause of their accumulation. Early in the course of DLB, vivid visual hallucinations are common. These hallucinations may occur simultaneously with mild movement disorder symptoms that may suggest Parkinson's disease, such as slowing of movements and muscular rigidity. Memory problems eventually become evident, but they may not be very dramatic early in the illness—and certainly not as dramatic as vivid visual hallucinations.

Yet another group of cognitive disorders seen by psychiatrists is called "frontotemporal dementias." The name comes from the fact that certain areas of the brain—parts of the frontal lobe and parts of the temporal lobe—are strongly affected in this group of disorders. Although memory, thinking, and speech eventually deteriorate in these disorders, the earliest signs are often major changes in personality. A person's behavior becomes increasingly inappropriate until family members won't go out with the person for fear that he or she may say or do very embarrassing things. For example, previously upstanding individuals with frontotemporal dementia may approach strangers and tell dirty jokes. They may make rude and inappropriate comments. They may exhibit substantial changes in their sex drive. Speech changes are also common in this form of cognitive disorder.

Little is known about the causes of frontotemporal dementias. However, recent research indicates that some forms of frontotemporal dementia may represent one of a group of disorders called "tauopathies," based on the fact that they involve abnormal collections of a protein called "*tau*" that makes up the cellular "backbone" of neurons. Abnormal accumulation of the *tau* protein may lead to the death of nerve cells. Recently, abnormalities of proteins other than *tau* have been shown to be involved in some types of frontotemporal dementias. Other than patient education about these disorders, effective treatments for frontotemporal dementias don't exist. Because dramatic changes in personality are sometimes the earliest symptom of the illness, psychiatrists are likely to be consulted in this disorder.

The cognitive disorders we have just discussed are illnesses that start gradually and progress slowly, meaning that full manifestation of the disorders takes months to years. They are related to brain deterioration (neurodegeneration). One last cognitive disorder is a bit different, however. Although it also influences thinking and behavior, its onset is more sudden and, in many cases, it may be reversible. This disorder is called delirium.

Delirium is a disorder (or more likely a group of disorders) in which something knocks the brain out of equilibrium. That "something" may be a subtle infection, overmedication with various therapeutic drugs, abnormal blood chemistries, adjustments following surgery, or the result of organ failure elsewhere in the body. Using an analogy to computers, we could say that delirium is something like the brain "crashing." This usually, but not always, occurs fairly quickly over hours or days. People become confused and are often disoriented, not knowing where they are, what day or time it is, and sometimes who they are. Their attention frequently drifts. Their short-term memory is impaired. Consciousness may wax and wane, ranging from somnolence to hypervigilance. Frequently, the brain plays tricks on afflicted individuals, and hallucinations, delusions, and illusions may occur. An *illusion* is a misinterpretation of a sensory input. For instance, a person suffering from a delirium may interpret light coming through the blinds as the flashbulb of a camera. Fluctuations in symptoms are very common. At times, the person may appear almost normal, but at other times during the same day quite impaired. Delirium can be quite dramatic and frightening to families. As with the dementing illnesses, family members may think the patient is "putting them on" or making things up. It is only when the marked confusion and agitation set in that the altered brain state becomes readily apparent.

Because hallucinations, delusions, agitation, and confusion are involved, psychiatrists are often consulted in the care of delirious patients. In fact, delirium is one of the most frequent reasons for psychiatric consults in a general medical hospital; in our experience, as many as one in three psychiatric consults in a general hospital is for delirium. The psychiatrist's role is to make the diagnosis of a delirium, help with the management of disruptive behaviors, and help the referring doctor begin the hunt for the cause. When the underlying cause is identified and corrected, the delirium may reverse. If left untreated, it can be fatal. If, however, the delirium is caused by an irreversible illness such as terminal kidney failure, the primary illness (in this example, the kidney failure) will progress, and the delirium is one of the symptoms suggesting that coma and death are approaching. Delirium is a medical and psychiatric emergency.

Personality Disorders

Personality disorders represent one of the most complicated and, for nonpsy-chiatrists, most misunderstood and frustrating areas in the field. The term *personality* refers to enduring aspects of our selves that flavor how we think and feel about others and our world. Our personalities reflect the ways our minds process information emotionally and cognitively. All of us inherit pre-dispositions that determine how we function, and these inherited predisposi-tions are shaped in response to the environments in which we develop. Our personalities have multiple dimensions. Psychologists often talk about these dimensions in terms of our tendencies to be open, conscientious, extroverted, agreeable, and anxious. Some psychiatrists, like C. Robert Cloninger, have championed other ways of thinking about personality based on temperament and character. The term *temperament* refers to underlying tendencies that govern how we usually respond to things that happen to us. It has four components reflecting how much we (1) are drawn to try new things, (2) are motivated by rewards and the approval of others, (3) take risks, and (4) are persistent in our goals and activities. *Character* traits reflect how much we are self-starters, cooperate with others, and understand that there is a world beyond ourselves and our own needs and that we are connected to that world. Certain aspects of these personality traits are inherited and the traits are ultimately shaped by the environment, particularly the environment in which we grow up. Together, they play a big role in making us who we are and in determining how we view others and how others view us.

As the name implies, personality disorders represent problems in tempera-ment and character and are probably most simply defined as "persistent and repeatedly maladaptive patterns of behavior." According to Cloninger, prob-lems in character, particularly problems in self-directedness and cooperative-ness, are fundamental defects in these disorders, and a person's underlying temperament drives the form the personality problem takes. Individuals with personality disorders are typically seen by others as being self-centered and having little concern about how their actions and words affect others. While they may show some interests in others, these interests are typically shallow and usually motivated by their own concerns. The behaviors associated with personality disorders are long-standing and are maladaptive in relation to others and the environment. Individuals with personality disorders have a lot of trouble getting along with people and are fairly rigid, tending to behave in repeated patterns that reflect how they view themselves and the world. Most times these individuals don't take personal responsibility for their problems. In effect, they repeatedly approach life from the perspective that "if you have a problem with what I do or say, that is your problem, not mine." This approach to life almost always begins in childhood or adolescence and persists into adulthood. Typically, the thinking and behaviors can be quite stereotyped (meaning that the individual has a tendency to apply a similar approach to all problems; for example, if being verbally abusive in one situation gets attention, then being verbally abusive in other situations will likely get the desired outcomes). Importantly, while personality disorders are distinct from the primary psychiatric disorders previously discussed, they clearly influence the outcome of major psychiatric disorders, including their response to treatment.

Categorizing personality disorders is a complex problem. DSM-IV considers them as categorical diagnoses, meaning that they are discrete disorders, distinct from other disorders. An alternative view proposes that defects in personality are "dimensions" that intersect with and flavor other psychiatric disorders. For example, major depression in a person who has no underlying personality problem will likely be different from major depression in a person who is persistently verbally abusive toward others. Depression tends to make underlying personality traits worse—and having lots of bad traits to begin with can be bad news in the context of depression. Perhaps reflecting the uncertainty in the field about personality disorders, DSM-IV codes them on a separate axis of diagnosis, referring to them as "Axis II disorders." In contrast, mood, anxiety, substance abuse, and psychotic disorders are called "Axis I disorders."

DSM-IV groups personality disorders in three clusters: an odd (or eccentric) group, a dramatic and volatile group, and an anxious and needy group. The odd cluster includes three diagnoses. The first diagnosis describes persons who exhibit persistently odd thinking, including magical ideas about the world. These individuals also exhibit cognitive and perceptual abnormalities, for example, illusions (misinterpreting sensations) and odd superstitions. Individuals with these types of symptoms are called "schizotypal personalities." The second diagnosis in the odd cluster describes individuals with "schizoid personalities": that is, persons that exhibit marked aloofness and withdrawal from social contacts. These persons prefer being alone to the company of others and are uncomfortable around other people. The third diagnosis in the eccentric group describes persons who have "paranoid personalities": They are hypersensitive to being around others and are suspicious and distrustful of them. All the persons with disorders in this cluster have detached and problematic interpersonal relationships. Some of the traits sound a lot like schizophrenia, but the persons with these personality disorders do not have the frank psychotic thinking, speech, or behavior seen in schizophrenia. These eccentric personalities do tend to run in the same families as persons with schizophrenia, so there may be overlap in genetics and other causes.

Patients with the second cluster of personality disorders are commonly encountered in psychiatric practices and are best described as dramatic and excessively emotional individuals who have a lot of difficulties in their interpersonal relationships. In fact, intense but unstable relationships may be one of the most defining features. Personality disorders in this cluster have been grouped into four categories, describing (1) individuals with blatant disregard for the rights of others as exhibited by criminal, deviant, and violent behaviors ("antisocial personalities"); (2) individuals who display excessive emotion and overly dramatic complaints about their symptoms and lives ("histrionic personalities"); (3) individuals who overemphasize their own self-worth and self-interests ("narcissistic personalities"); and (4) a dramatically unstable and impulsive group that is difficult to define ("borderline personalities"). Borderline personality disorder occurs more often in women than in men and is characterized by very volatile and at times abusive interpersonal relationships. Persons with this disorder also report a large number of dramatic psychiatric symptoms that can include impulsive and repeated bouts of self-harm (wrist cutting, self-mutilation, and intentional overdoses of medications). The term *borderline* derives from older psychiatric concepts that viewed the severity of symptoms in these persons as bordering on psychosis, reflecting the fact that they can have episodes that appear to be psychotic or at least markedly disturbed to outside observers. These individuals tend to see the world in black and white—people are either all good or all bad—and how they view others can change rapidly depending on whether the others are doing what those with borderline personality want them to do at the time.

Several of these dramatic personality syndromes—borderline, histrionic, and perhaps antisocial—appear to overlap with what is called "somatoform disorders." These disorders are characterized by symptoms that tend to mimic medical conditions but that have no adequate medical explanation. The overlap may be most evident with "somatization disorder" (Briquet's syndrome), a distinct somatoform disorder that was previously known as "hysteria." Individuals with somatization disorder report a large number of unexplained, sometimes dramatic medical symptoms and tend to see many doctors and to have many medical procedures. They can also have a large number of psychiatric symptoms that are hard to classify, much like persons with borderline personality disorder. In some clinical studies, the overlap between borderline personality disorder and somatization disorder is substantial, indicating that they may be different manifestations of the same underlying dysfunction.

Individuals with any of these dramatic personality disorders can be very difficult to deal with and treat. They can also develop Axis I psychiatric disorders, particularly mood and substance abuse disorders, and in many cases it can be very difficult to determine where the boundary between the Axis I disorder and the personality disorder lies. These individuals can also be very frustrating for families and friends because they can be demanding, manipulative, and volatile. At other times, they can be charming and engaging. In other words, they tend to run "hot and cold," like a "Dr. Jekyll and Mr. Hyde." Because of their volatility, some individuals with these dramatic personality disorders are diagnosed with bipolar disorder and its milder versions (like bipolar II disorder or cyclothymic disorder). In the absence of symptoms of unequivocal mania, the bipolar diagnosis is largely inappropriate and can result in excessive and ineffective treatment with numerous psychiatric medications. That these patients often engage in substance abuse can also confuse the picture, particularly when stimulants (cocaine, amphetamines) or psychosis-inducing drugs (PCP) are involved.

The third cluster of personality disorders is characterized by chronic anxiety, fear, and neediness. These disorders describe persons who are socially inhibited and avoid others because of fears of rejection ("avoidant personalities"), are overly submissive to and dependent upon others for help and care ("dependent personalities"), and are perfectionistic, rigid, and controlling ("obsessive-compulsive personalities"). In the latter case, the distinction between obsessive-compulsive personality disorder and the Axis I diagnosis of obsessive-compulsive disorder (OCD) at times can be difficult. Individuals with this cluster of personality disorders, particularly the dependent personalities, tend to be "passive aggressive." That is, their apparent incompetence and ineffectiveness in activities and relationships are a way of manipulating, getting back at, and controlling family, friends, caregivers, and employers. Passive-aggressive behavior is not specific to this cluster of disorders, however, and can be seen across a range of personality problems.

Presently, we understand little about the biological mechanisms underlying the personality disorders. However, efforts aimed at understanding human emotional, motivational, and cognitive processing are likely to pay dividends because defects in emotional regulation and social cognition appear to be important in these disorders, particularly in the dramatic group. Treatment of individuals with personality disorders is usually very difficult, and improvement in symptoms is slow to occur. There are no clearly effective treatments that improve personality. Generally, treatment with psychiatric medications is focused on concurrent depression and substance abuse disorders. Various forms of psychotherapy focused on defining expectations and setting limits for tolerated behaviors are very important in management, particularly in the dramatic cluster. The focus in therapy is on "here and now" problems and on the patients' responsibility for them, not on the long-standing strife that these individuals have encountered or on the reasons they feel they have been wronged by life. A key in the management of these individuals is to hold them responsible for their manipulative, volatile, and inappropriate behaviors. Often these patients and their families seek psychiatric attention and pressure for quick medication fixes for their problems. But there are no such quick fixes, and consistent "tough love" with emphasis on personal responsibility is one of the mainstays of management.

Adjustment Disorders

Persons suffering from adjustment disorders often come to the attention of mental health professionals and primary care physicians. This group of disorders is used to describe overwhelming and unhealthy psychological responses to typical life stressors. A person suffering from an adjustment disorder is considered to be having a response that is disproportionate to the nature of the stressor; that is, it exceeds the response that a typical person would have when exposed to the same stressor. The disorder also can apply to a person who is responding to a stressor in a manner that leads to significantly impaired function at work or school. The DSM-IV definition of adjustment disorders is designed to be distinct from that of post-traumatic stress disorder. In PTSD, the stressor is objectively severe and traumatic, one that would likely distress most people (e.g., a severe accident or physical assault). Also, in an adjustment disorder, the behavioral response (e.g., depressed mood) to the stressor is not accompanied by enough other symptoms to fulfill criteria for another major psychiatric diagnosis (e.g., a full-blown mood disorder such as major depression). Adjustment disorder diagnoses are accompanied by descriptors based on the predominant symptoms that the patient is exhibiting: for example, adjustment disorder with depressed mood, or adjustment disorder with anxiety.

An example of someone with an adjustment disorder might be a young woman who responds to the breakup of a relationship with gestures of self-harm, such as scratching her arm with a razor blade. This action might lead the young woman's family to bring her to the emergency room for an evaluation of suicidal intent. In the emergency room, the young woman may report that she felt fine until the previous night when her boyfriend broke up with her and she became overwhelmed and sad. Now, she feels embarrassed by her response (cutting herself) and indicates that she had no intent to end her life. As one might surmise, adjustment disorders may be influenced by the individual's coping skills, which can be a reflection of his or her underlying personality.

Because of the wide range of conditions that may be associated with an adjustment disorder and the possibility that it can be the early manifestation of another psychiatric disorder, such as major depression or panic disorder, it is important that mental health professionals carefully and repeatedly evaluate a person who initially fulfills criteria for an adjustment disorder. Treatment of adjustment disorders usually consists of brief individual or group psychotherapy with a mental health professional. If the stressor was a one-time event, the adjustment disorder usually resolves quickly. In fact, if the symptoms last for more than three months following a single stressor, then the diagnosis should be reconsidered. At times, it can be difficult to distinguish an adjustment disorder from mood or anxiety disorders; this can sometimes lead to unnecessary and long-term treatment with psychiatric medications. Brief treatment with medications can sometimes be helpful (e.g., to relieve acute anxiety or help with sleep), but the primary treatment approach for adjustment disorders is usually psychological intervention coupled with close follow-up to make sure that a longer-term psychiatric disorder does not develop.

Other Disorders

The disorders discussed in this chapter reflect the most common problems diagnosed and treated by general psychiatrists. There are, however, several other categories of psychiatric disorders that should be mentioned. Eating disorders are complex disorders marked by problems with food intake and body weight. They are particularly prevalent among young women and can be life threatening. Anorexia nervosa is characterized by persistent problems with body image and a rigid desire to be thin, often to the point of starvation. Bulimia nervosa is characterized by repeated bouts of binge eating and "purging" (vomiting and overuse of laxatives). Eating disorders, like personality disorders, are difficult to treat. Most effective strategies deal with concomitant problems such as depression and substance use, including laxative abuse. Engaging the family in treatment is an important component of dealing with these disorders.

Psychiatrists are sometimes involved in diagnosing and managing individuals with a variety of sexual problems. These include gender identity disorders (previously referred to as "transexualism"), sexual dysfunctions, and paraphilias (sexual deviations). These problems are typically not common in general psychiatric practices but are areas of specialized interest for some psychiatrists. General psychiatrists can play important roles in helping to determine whether other psychiatric disorders are contributing to sexual problems, particularly those involving sexual drive and performance. Some specially trained psychiatrists (called forensic psychiatrists) who work at the interface of psychiatry and the law may be involved in the evaluation and treatment of individuals who exhibit sexual deviations and criminal behavior.

Other important groups of disorders occur in children and adolescents and include autism and attention deficit hyperactivity disorder, among others. These are becoming increasingly recognized as major problems in the United States, but they are beyond the scope of this book and our areas of expertise. Again, readers are referred to general textbooks of psychiatry and DSM-IV for information about these disorders.

Take-Home Messages

- Psychiatric disorders are diagnosed using specific criteria that are evolving as more is discovered about the disorders. The reliability for most major psychiatric diagnoses is very high, in many cases matching or exceeding the reliability of medical and neurological diagnoses. The validity of psychiatric diagnoses as discrete disease entities has been more difficult to establish. However, the major diagnoses have a good deal of clinical utility for determining appropriate treatment courses and communication among health professionals.

- Psychiatrists commonly care for patients with mood, anxiety, psychotic, substance abuse, cognitive, and personality disorders. Mood disorders, particularly depression in its various forms, represent the bulk of many psychiatrists' practices.

- Personality disorders represent complex, long-standing problems with temperament, character, and emotional regulation. Importantly, persons with these disorders are not frankly psychotic and are difficult to treat effectively. The complex nature of these disorders can lead to the inappropriate use of multiple psychiatric medications; the benefits of such treatment are not clear. Psychotherapeutic approaches that emphasize patients' responsibility for their problems and that set limits on manipulative and inappropriate behavior are very important in management. There are no quick fixes for the personality disorders.

···three···

Warning Signs

What are the early signs of a psychiatric disorder? How can a person recognize early symptoms of a relapse of a preexisting illness? What symptoms should lead someone to seek psychiatric care? Psychiatrists are asked these questions regularly, often by people who are concerned about the behavior of a friend or family member. Some psychiatric disorders are associated with loss of insight, and those afflicted by these illnesses may accept changes in their thinking, mood, and behavior as "normal" or "understandable" under the circumstances of their lives. It frequently falls to friends and family members to recognize that something is wrong and to encourage the person to seek help. In this chapter, we will discuss warning signs that indicate that an individual has or may be developing a serious psychiatric disorder. The features discussed here do not represent a complete list of warning signs of every psychiatric disorder we've discussed so far or of the complications (e.g., risk of suicide or violence) that are sometimes associated with many of these illnesses. Rather, these signs represent some typical red flags that indicate that psychiatric evaluation may be warranted. Family and friends should be especially vigilant for warning signs of relapsing illness when a person is decreasing or discontinuing treatment. Far too often, patients decide they are doing well and elect to stop treatments, including discontinuing their medications. If this decision is premature, symptoms can return within days, weeks, or months.

Some mental disorders develop gradually. For example, the low mood or anxiety associated with major depression and certain anxiety disorders can creep up on individuals and go unrecognized for weeks or months. In contrast, symptoms of mania or acute psychosis can appear suddenly and dramatically—even the most casual observer can recognize that something is terribly wrong. Other psychiatric symptoms, like those associated with panic attacks, are dramatic but can be confused with medical or neurological problems. It is important to recognize when a *change* has occurred in a person's thinking, motivation, or emotions and to know when these changes indicate the possibility of serious psychiatric problems.

It will become evident in this chapter that various warning signs are not necessarily specific to one category of illness. For example, withdrawn behavior is associated with several psychiatric disorders, including depression, schizophrenia, obsessive-compulsive disorder, dementia, or other conditions. Similarly, changes in sleep patterns may be involved in numerous psychiatric or medical disorders.

Warning Signs of Depressive Disorders

Several behavioral changes associated with the presence of a clinically significant depression warrant psychiatric evaluation. Warning signs include the following:

- Persistent sadness lasting several weeks or more. Particularly when combined with spontaneous crying spells or changes in a person's ability to function at home or at work, sadness often marks the beginning of a depressive episode or relapse of a previous episode.
- Persistent sullenness, moodiness, and irritability.
- Social withdrawal. Some individuals who are developing a depression begin to isolate themselves from friends and family; they lose interest in activities that they previously enjoyed, including sex and hobbies.
- Absenteeism from, or the inability to function at, work or school.
- Sleep difficulties, including problems with falling and/or staying asleep. Awakening in the early morning hours without the ability to fall back to sleep is a classic feature of depression.
- Unintentional changes in appetite accompanied by either weight loss or weight gain.
- Recurrent thoughts about death in an otherwise healthy individual, including suicidal thoughts.

It is important to remember that everyone has bad days now and then; however, *persistent* changes in one or more of the above-mentioned behaviors should alert family and friends that something may be wrong and that the person exhibiting such symptoms should be seen by a mental health professional.

Suicidal Thoughts and Behavior

Suicide is one of the most devastating complications of psychiatric illness and is associated with many psychiatric disorders, including mood disorders, substance abuse disorders, psychotic disorders, some anxiety disorders, and some personality disorders, particularly those complicated by major depression or substance abuse. All suicidal thinking and behavior, including suicidal gestures (e.g., relatively minor drug overdoses or minor wrist cuttings), must be taken seriously and require careful evaluation. Suicidal gestures without intent to die are frequently symptoms of personality disorders, and these "cries for help" require careful diagnosis, brief interventions, and in some cases, longer-term psychiatric care.

Many people have the notion that asking someone whether he or she is suicidal can "plant the idea" in that person's mind. There is absolutely no evidence that this is true. In fact, most patients with suicidal thoughts are relieved to have the opportunity to talk openly about them and to share the burden they have been carrying. They will often initially communicate their thinking to others in an indirect fashion. Comments such as "I'd be better off dead" or "you won't have to worry about dealing with me much longer" are statements that should raise concern, particularly when they represent a change in behavior and occur in the context of other psychiatric symptoms. Similarly, indications that the person doesn't expect to be around for an upcoming event are potentially important warning signs. Expressions of worthlessness, hopelessness, and helplessness should also raise concern. For family and friends, such comments might be best handled by suggesting that the individual see a doctor or seek psychiatric care.

Individuals with suicidal ideas are particularly at risk when they are intoxicated with drugs or alcohol. Many abused drugs adversely affect mood, either during the period of intoxication or as the intoxication winds down. Thus, threats of suicide during intoxication are of major concern, in part because inhibitions and normal constraints on behavior are relaxed by the intoxicated state. This is clearly the case among alcoholics. Alcoholics carry increased suicide risk compared to the general population, and they are at greatest risk for suicide when they are drunk. Additionally, alcoholics are at greater risk of suicide at times when they have experienced significant recent losses in relationships, jobs, or finances. Threats, dire conversations, and increased drinking during such periods must be taken very seriously.

All suicidal thoughts, gestures, or attempts should be evaluated psychiatrically. Sometimes these suicidal feelings may indicate a significant depression or other major mental disorder. Sometimes they may be an impulsive reaction to life circumstances or a reflection of a person's personality. In all cases, however, the potential for eventual harm is significant. Although it is not possible to prevent every suicide, mental health professionals can help decrease the risk or delay this tragic outcome. In many cases, a delay is all that is needed for patients to reconsider their actions.

Warning Signs of Anxiety Disorders

Symptoms of anxiety disorders typically produce significant discomfort, and individuals often recognize that something is wrong. They may not recognize, however, that the symptoms need psychiatric attention. For example, panic attacks are discrete and dramatic events that can lead a person to believe she or he is having a "nervous breakdown" or heart attack. This often prompts a visit to an emergency room or a primary care doctor. Other anxiety symptoms, like obsessions, may go unrecognized as being manifestations of a psychiatric disorder. In such instances, individuals may be viewed as overly cautious and meticulous, traits that can be beneficial in some situations and that are not necessarily signs of illness. However, the presence of ritualistic compulsions (e.g., counting rituals, repeatedly checking locks, or making sure that one's clothes and possessions are kept in precise order) can be signs of obsessive-compulsive disorder, particularly when the compulsions are rigidly pursued and met with irritability or marked anxiety when preempted. Other rituals, such as repeated showering during a single day or repeated hand washing, should be sufficient to prompt concern from family and friends. Compulsive hoarding is another trait that should prompt concern. Some degree of nervousness and worrying may be appropriate, but when an individual worries to such a degree that it consistently interferes with work and social interactions, then family and friends might consider encouraging the person to be evaluated for the possibility of having a generalized anxiety disorder.

When an individual has experienced a major life-threatening event (e.g., a severe accident or injury), it is possible that he or she may develop post-traumatic stress disorder (PTSD). Most individuals experience some anxiety and/or depressive symptoms after such events but do not go on to full-blown PTSD. Based on studies of survivors of major disasters, it appears that individuals who begin to avoid their usual activities and exhibit numbness toward their experience and those around them are at increased risk for developing persistent PTSD.

Warning Signs of Psychosis

Full-blown psychotic disorders are relatively easy to detect. Most people readily recognize acutely agitated, bizarre, and disruptive behavior when they see it. Recognizing the early and more subtle changes that can accompany such illnesses as schizophrenia, psychotic major depression, or bipolar disorder can be much more problematic, however. Early warning signs may include:

- A significant change in an individual's sleep-wake cycle. Individuals often develop noticeable changes in their sleep patterns at the onset of psychotic disorders, particularly disorders that are accompanied by agitation. Dramatic changes in sleep, such as decreased need for sleep to the extent that a person starts staying up all night, are major warning signs. When sleep changes are accompanied by other changes in behavior, such as pacing about the house and talking to oneself or to persons others can't see, the level of concern should be very high. Similarly, when a person makes repeated, unexpected phone calls to others in the middle of the night, it can be an indication of a serious problem, particularly when the content of the calls doesn't make a lot of sense or consists of unsubstantiated claims (e.g., that someone is spying on or trying to harm the individual).

- Conspicuous changes in a person's speech. These may include speech that is very rapid and difficult to interrupt, that is digressive and wanders from topic to topic, or that is completely incomprehensible.

- Troubling content in the individual's speech. For example, the individual may voice concern about being poisoned, being the victim of a conspiracy, or being targeted by some major organization such as the police, CIA, federal government, or mafia. Or the individual may claim to have developed special powers (e.g., telepathy or the ability to control the stock market) or to have been chosen by their god or government to do special things.

- Social withdrawal. Some individuals become increasingly withdrawn and refuse to interact with others when they are becoming psychotic, and therefore they don't readily describe their thinking or concerns to others.

All of these features are potential warning signs of an existing or impending psychotic disorder and indicate a need for psychiatric evaluation.

Violent Behavior

Statistically speaking, violent acts are rare occurrences in the general population and thus are rare in patients with psychiatric disorders. Nonetheless, such patients, particularly those with psychotic disorders, have an increased chance of either committing or being the victim of a violent act. Some of this increased risk is a result of the chaotic lifestyles sometimes associated with psychotic illnesses, particularly those complicated by substance abuse. For persons with antisocial personality disorder (sociopathy), violence can be part of a life-long pattern of behavior. For such individuals, drugs of abuse may make their violent tendencies worse. In fact, all violent behavior is made worse by substance use and abuse.

Psychiatrists are often asked to make predictions about the likelihood of violence in individuals with psychiatric disorders. This can be extremely difficult, and the tendency is to err on the side of caution, particularly when the concerns are raised in the context of a major psychiatric disorder. Sometimes, this means evaluating the person in a protected environment (hospital) for a few days.

The best predictor of the risk for future violence is a past history of violence. For example, one must be extremely careful when a psychiatrically ill patient with a past history of violence is making threats or appears agitated and irritable. Warning signs can include the person becoming outraged over little things or taking major offense to seemingly harmless comments. Agitated behavior (e.g., pacing, exaggerated startle responses, and threatening gestures), particularly in the context of intoxication with drugs or alcohol, is also a major warning sign. Persons who become violent when intoxicated are at substantial risk of violence if they continue abusing alcohol or other drugs. Alcohol and other drugs of abuse are associated with at least half of all homicides in the United States.

When an illness such as schizophrenia or bipolar disorder is contributing to a person's violent tendencies, psychiatrists frequently are involved in the person's treatment. On the other hand, when the violence is related to a life-long pattern of antisocial behavior, the criminal justice system, and not the mental health system, often becomes involved.

Warning Signs of Substance Abuse

Noticeable changes in behavior can be the first signs that an individual is having problems with substance abuse. Warning signs may include:

- Changes in sleep-wake patterns (including reversed sleep-wake cycles and keeping odd hours).

- Inattention to usual habits and poor self-care (in personal hygiene, cleanliness, clothing).

- Changes in performance at school or work, including recurrent problems with absenteeism.

- Problems with concentration, slurred speech, and impaired coordination.

- The obvious smell of an abused drug (e.g., alcohol or marijuana) on the individual.

- The amount of a substance such as alcohol that an individual consumes. Some studies indicate that episodes of consuming four or more alcohol-containing drinks in a day constitute "at risk" drinking. This doesn't mean that a substance abuse disorder is necessarily present, but rather that this degree of alcohol consumption puts the individual at risk for complications from drinking (e.g., car accidents and traffic violations, interpersonal conflicts, and problems at work).

- Periods of irritability and mood swings can accompany alternating episodes of intoxication, hangover, and withdrawal.

Family, friends, and physicians often overlook early signs of substance abuse. By the time the problem is openly recognized, significant personal, interpersonal, and perhaps legal repercussions may already have occurred. Families can help by talking with their loved ones about undergoing a psychiatric or medical evaluation. Some persons exhibiting signs of substance abuse do have enough insight to take this advice, especially when interpersonal relationships and job performance are starting to be influenced adversely by the behavioral changes.

Warning Signs of Personality Disorders

Personality disorders are relatively common, and we have all encountered people with these disorders in a variety of settings, including work, school, and other social situations. The behaviors associated with personality disorders are long-standing, typically dating to a person's adolescence, so recognizing a change in a person's behavior is not usually the issue. Hallmarks of personality disorders include the following:

- A repeated pattern of manipulative interpersonal interactions. Such individuals often try, for example, to get other people to do their work for them, and they repeatedly cite vague physical symptoms or life circumstances to get out of obligations and elicit sympathy from others. These individuals are sometimes popularly referred to as "drama queens" (and "kings"). They also commonly use passive-aggressive behavior to control others, for example, by being unable to perform certain tasks because of relatively minor physical problems or purposeful ineptness.

- A profound sense of martyrly persecution, a sense of having been wronged by life and misunderstood and mistreated by others (e.g., bosses, co-workers, and family members).

- In some cases, extremely volatile and disruptive behavior that is often used to control others and social situations. Such individuals appear to run "hot and cold," quickly switching their outlook from everything being good to everything being miserable, and in the process involving those around them in these mood swings.

- Suicidal behaviors, including minor overdoses of medications or bouts of wrist cutting and self-mutilation. As noted previously, these episodes of self-harm are at times "cries for help" and may require psychiatric hospitalization; at other times, these episodes are forms of manipulation.

- Problems with depression and substance abuse, which often make symptoms of the personality disorder worse and greatly increase the risk of completed suicide.

These patterns of behavior, especially if they are persistent and interfere with a person's daily function, warrant an evaluation by a mental health professional.

Warning Signs of Delirium or Dementia

Most of us over the age of 50 have occasionally forgotten a name or experienced other momentary blips in memory recall. Such occasional "senior moments" usually do not indicate that we are developing an illness. Moreover, most people find it more difficult to multi-task as they age, and this too is not unusual. Given enough time, even people in their 80s or 90s can complete complex tasks, and their reading, organizational, and math skills can hold their own as long as they aren't rushed. However, for people of all ages, signs of mental deterioration—such as marked confusion, especially with sudden onset—are not normal and should be evaluated medically. Confusion can result from a variety of causes ranging from a stroke to abnormal sugar levels to a variety of other medical and neurological disorders to problems resulting from the medications used to treat these conditions. Rapid changes in mental status usually indicate that something is seriously wrong with brain function and are warning signs that should not be ignored.

More subtle and gradually progressive changes in memory, judgment, orientation, and organizational skills can be harder to detect. Most critical are changes that begin to interfere significantly with a person's ability to complete everyday tasks. Such changes might include, for example, the *frequent* forgetting of names coupled with difficulties in keeping one's checkbook up to date and in knowing how much change to get at the supermarket checkout. These may suggest the beginning of a dementing illness and should be evaluated by a physician. Primary care physicians are accustomed to evaluating such cognitive changes, although psychiatrists and neurologists have specialized expertise in these areas.

Take-Home Messages

- In some cases, the onset of a psychiatric disorder is relatively sudden and obvious to everyone. More often, however, the onset is subtle and involves gradual changes in behavior, thinking, and daily routine. Recognizing these changes can be difficult, but alterations in sleep-wake cycles, appetite, personal hygiene, and interpersonal interactions are common.

- For most people, major depression and substance abuse disorders will be the most common psychiatric disorders they encounter.

Less common but no less devastating are psychotic disorders. Recognizing early signs and symptoms of all of these disorders can go a long way toward helping people with these disorders get appropriate help early in the course of an episode of illness.

- Identifying the psychiatric problems of people with personality disorders is less about recognizing changes in their behavior or thinking than about recognizing how the existing core symptoms of these disorders interfere with the everyday lives of these individuals and others around them. If you feel that you are being used or manipulated in your interpersonal interactions with someone, you may well be dealing with a person with a personality disorder. Psychiatric evaluation is warranted especially if this individual exhibits behavior that is disruptive or dangerous or otherwise interferes with his or her function.

- Suicide and violence are complications of major psychiatric disorders. Fortunately, these are rare events from a statistical standpoint. Nonetheless, caution should be exercised with individuals who are talking openly about their death or making dire predictions about their future. The majority of persons who commit suicide communicate their intent at some point. Similarly, extreme caution should be exercised with individuals who are agitated or threatening, particularly those with a prior history of violence. In the case of suicidal and violent behavior, highest risk is associated with those who are psychotic or intoxicated with drugs or alcohol.

- The rapid onset of mental confusion requires urgent medical attention. Gradually progressing changes in memory, thinking, and organizational skills that occur over several months or more or that begin to interfere with everyday function should also be brought to a doctor's attention.

···*four*···

Who Are Psychiatrists and What Do They Actually Do?

This chapter is about psychiatrists themselves—about how they are trained and how their training clearly distinguishes them from other mental health professionals, such as clinical psychologists or social workers, and prepares them for their practice as physicians who specialize in the diagnosis and treatment of mental disorders. We will also describe the nature of that practice and the various challenges and complications that psychiatrists encounter in the care of patients with psychiatric illness. In other words, because there is considerable misunderstanding in the general public, including among many patients and families, about the role that psychiatrists play in the mental health world, we believe it will be helpful to describe in some detail who they are and what they do.

Psychiatrists Are Medical Doctors with Specialty Training

Like other doctors, psychiatrists have attended medical school where they spent four years learning about the normal and abnormal function of the human body. In medical school, the education of future psychiatrists is no different from that of medical students who become internists or surgeons. In the United States, medical school is typically preceded by a four-year undergraduate education in which all future physicians ("pre-meds") are required to follow a rigorous scientific program that includes core courses in chemistry, physics, biology, and certain types of mathematics. Once they enter medical school, all students are required to take preclinical courses dealing with the "basic sciences," including anatomy (the structure of the human body), normal and abnormal human physiology (how the body works), pharmacology (how medications and other drugs work on the body), and pathology (changes in bodily tissues caused by illness), among others. Study of the basic sciences is complemented by clinical training, during which all medical students take core courses with direct patient experience in internal medicine, surgery, pediatrics, obstetrics and gynecology, neurology, and psychiatry, as well as certain subspecialty areas. They also take elective courses in areas of particular interest. Importantly for consumers, no other mental health professional receives the intensive medical training described here—and this is only the beginning.

Upon graduation from medical school, students receive their medical doctor, or MD, degree. It is at this point that the new MDs pursue in-depth training in the specialty of their choice. Those interested in psychiatry take part in training that focuses on disorders of the human mind and behavior. This post-medical school period is referred to as "residency training," just as it is for other branches of medicine. For general psychiatrists, residency training lasts four years. The first year usually includes at least four months of clinical experience in general internal medicine, two or more months in neurology, and several months in psychiatry. During their internal medicine and neurology rotations, psychiatry residents treat patients who are acutely ill with medical and neurological illnesses, working side by side with residents who are training to become internists and neurologists under the careful supervision of specialists in these fields.

The remainder of the four years of residency largely focuses on mental disorders and includes both coursework (didactics) in specific topics, such as interviewing skills, psychopharmacology, and psychotherapy, and extensive hands-on experience with patients. Psychiatric training is conducted in a variety of hospital and outpatient settings where residents are exposed to a broad range of mental illnesses. Training focuses heavily on understanding the diagnosis, treatment, and outcome of mental disorders primarily in adults, with some exposure to the same concerns as they relate to children and adolescents. Thus, among mental health professionals, only psychiatrists receive this type of detailed education in medical, neurological, and mental disorders.

To ensure quality, psychiatric residency programs are certified by the Accreditation Council for Graduate Medical Education (ACGME). In order to gain certification, programs must demonstrate that they provide rigorous educational experiences that include broad exposure to a variety of psychiatric diagnoses and treatment modalities over a broad age range of patients. Following successful completion of a four-year general residency program, psychiatrists are eligible to seek "board certification" through the American Board of Psychiatry and Neurology (ABPN). This board certification is one marker of quality among psychiatrists, at least as defined by the ability to pass a complex examination that includes both written and oral portions. To practice psychiatry in the United States, psychiatrists must have a medical license issued by their state board of healing arts, but they do *not* have to have ABPN certification. Thus, consumers should be aware that not all psychiatrists carry the stamp of board certification.

The educational path just described is typical for general psychiatrists. Some psychiatrists, however, acquire additional intensive training in specific areas of interest. These include child and adolescent psychiatry, geriatric psychiatry, forensic (legal) psychiatry, addiction psychiatry, and consultation-liaison (CL) psychiatry; in this latter subspecialty, psychiatrists work with patients who have complex medical and surgical illnesses and interact closely with physicians in many other clinical specialties. These subspecialty training programs are usually one or two years in duration, and separate board certification is available in these areas. While at first glance, the additional training would seem to be valuable, there is some controversy about the added benefits of pursuing certification in certain subspecialties, given that general psychiatrists are usually well equipped, after eight years of training (four years of medical school and four years of psychiatry residency), to deal with the broad range of psychiatric disorders. Nonetheless, such subspecialty training has become increasingly recognized as necessary to adequately address the particular complexities involved in these subgroups or areas of practice. In child and adolescent psychiatry, for example, additional training is in essence mandatory because of the complexities of childhood and adolescent development and the different types of disorders seen in these age groups (e.g., autism, mental retardation, attention deficit hyperactivity disorder, and so on). Similarly, forensic psychiatrists work in a difficult area involving the interface between mental disorders and the legal system and benefit greatly from additional training that extends beyond the usual psychiatric education. Some psychiatrists also seek further training in specific forms of psychotherapy (talk therapy), neuropsychiatry (the interface between neurology, neuropsychology, and psychiatry), and other areas.

As is true of other physicians, all psychiatrists must participate in annual continuing medical education (CME) to maintain their licensure. This is one way that state boards ensure that physicians maintain skills relevant to their clinical disciplines. Additionally, the ABPN now requires recertification for most psychiatrists on a regular basis, and the recertification process includes rigorous CME exercises aimed at improving clinical practice.

The Psychiatric Examination of Patients

A psychiatrist's office is typically a bit different from the offices of other physicians. There are usually fewer or no areas for physical examination and laboratory tests and more space for meeting with patients and their families. Because a psychiatric examination is largely based on a focused conversation with the patient, the ability to conduct interviews in a relaxed and comfortable setting is important. Psychiatrists may also conduct at least parts of a physical examination, largely aimed at assessing neurological function (reflexes, sensation, balance, gait, and strength), when there is reason to suspect a neurologic condition. Some psychiatrists choose to do very little physical examination themselves, preferring to stick to their expertise in the "mental status examination," which focuses on evaluating the patient's emotional and cognitive function. We will describe how this evaluation is done in more detail shortly. Psychiatrists generally work in fairly close collaboration with other physicians involved in a patient's care, particularly primary care doctors, internists, and neurologists. The management of medical illnesses (e.g., diabetes, hypertension) is usually left to internists and primary care doctors while the psychiatrist concentrates on managing mental disorders. It is not unusual, however, for psychiatrists to spend considerable time helping patients to understand the nature of their medical disorders and the impact of these conditions on mental function.

The first visit to a psychiatrist usually involves an interview and examination lasting 30 to 90 minutes. The bulk of this time involves an in-depth meeting between the psychiatrist and the patient (and accompanying family members if the patient gives permission). The interview is based on questions and approaches that are similar to those used by other doctors, although a psychiatrist spends more time in this interview process. Psychiatrists receive considerable training in how to interview patients and their families and ask an array of questions to help patients describe their problems. Psychiatric diagnoses largely depend on the information elicited by these questions, rather than on laboratory studies, and thus facilitating dialogue with the patient is of critical importance. The questions can range from open ended (e.g., "can you tell me more about that?" or "how did that make you feel?") to more directed (e.g., "do you have trouble sleeping?" or "has your appetite changed?"). Because some issues dealt with in psychiatry are very sensitive and difficult for patients to talk about, psychiatrists will also use what are called "facilitating questions" to help normalize the thoughts and feelings that patients may have. For example, "when people are feeling low, they sometimes have thoughts about death and even think about killing themselves. . . . Have you ever had these types of thoughts?" The goal is to get patients to talk about their painful experiences and to help the psychiatrist understand how serious things have been.

During a psychiatric interview, a lot of time is spent exploring the reasons why a patient has sought psychiatric care, with major emphasis on the signs and symptoms associated with specific psychiatric disorders. This process includes numerous questions about mood, sleep, appetite, and activities, and about the patients' current state as it affects their overall ability to function at home and work. Specific questions also address whether a patient has unusual experiences like hallucinations (e.g., hearing voices when no one is around) or delusions (fixed false beliefs that are out of social context, such as believing that others are trying to poison the patient or control the patient's mind). A number of questions focus on areas of specific concern for psychiatrists, including suicidal ideas and behavior as well as potential for violence. Psychiatrists also ask about any history of alcohol or illicit drug use in considerable detail. Because psychiatric disorders have long-term courses in which symptoms can wax and wane over years, the psychiatrist often inquires in detail about how the patient's symptoms have changed over the years and whether any prior treatments have been beneficial. The more a patient understands his or her illness and can describe its past course, the better it is for both the psychiatrist and the patient.

Because psychiatric disorders can overlap with other medical and neurological conditions, patients can expect to be asked about nonpsychiatric disorders and their treatments, including allergies to any medications. Psychiatrists also focus a great deal on the social aspects of a patient's disorder, including childhood, education, jobs, marriages, and military service, probing for problems in any of these areas. Because psychiatric disorders tend to run in families and have a complex genetic basis, psychiatrists also ask a lot of questions about illnesses in a patient's family and their outcome.

Some parts of a psychiatric evaluation can seem strange to patients. Questions about "hearing voices" or about thoughts of suicide or homicide can seem especially odd to those patients who have never had these symptoms. Nonetheless, these are important parts of the examination. One of the more peculiar aspects of a psychiatric interview, at least for many patients, is the "sensorium and intellect" portion of a formal mental status examination. The term *sensorium* refers to people's perception of their environment (attention and orientation to time, place, and person) and *intellect* to the cognitive functions of their brain. In this part of the exam, the psychiatrist asks questions dealing with language (naming objects, repeating phrases), general intellect, attention, orientation (e.g., knowing the date, one's current location, and one's name), memory (recall of recent and remote information), simple calculations, and judgment (e.g., how the patient responds in social situations). Psychiatrists may also ask what some people jokingly refer to as "chicken-and-egg" questions that test the patient's ability to do higher-level abstract reasoning. Examples include questions such as "how are an apple and an orange alike?" or "what does the saying 'a stitch in time saves nine' mean?" Again, for patients with no defects in these spheres, the questions might seem strange, but they are very important for determining an individual's current intellectual state and overall neurological status.

Rating scales are increasingly being used in clinical practice in order to measure and follow symptoms. These rating scales include a variety of well-validated instruments for detecting and monitoring the symptoms of various mental disorders. Some scales are filled out by the patient ("self-report"), while others are administered by the physician or another member of the treatment team. One example is the Beck Depression Inventory (BDI), a self-report questionnaire that can be very helpful in monitoring the effectiveness of treatments for depression. Other examples include the Mini-Mental Status Examination (MMSE), which is a brief test used to monitor cognitive function, and the Abnormal Involuntary Movement Scale (AIMS), which is used to monitor the side effects of some medications. Other questionnaires are directed toward assessing anxiety, alcohol use, and other symptoms. These rating scales can be very helpful in providing "objective" data that psychiatrists (and other doctors) can integrate with global clinical impressions derived from their examination of the patient. Importantly, however, these instruments do not replace the critical role of the doctor–patient interaction in determining a patient's psychiatric condition and response to treatment.

Following the initial detailed examination, psychiatrists usually discuss with the patient the nature of the signs and symptoms they have observed. This leads to a discussion about likely diagnoses and treatment options. The treatment of psychiatric disorders, like all medical disorders, involves collaboration between the doctor and the patient. Thus, the psychiatrist usually discusses several options with the patient and gives recommendations for treatment. The nature of these treatments will be discussed later in the book, but in brief, they could include a variety of approaches ranging from forms of psychotherapy to medications and brain stimulation techniques (e.g., electroconvulsive therapy, or ECT). In severe cases, psychiatric hospitalization might be discussed. The option for no treatment at all is also possible and is usually discussed with the patient. A discussion of the potential risks and benefits of the various treatment options is also a part of the interview process. Risks include not only the potential side effects of treatment but also the potential complications of untreated illness.

Psychiatrists are a bit like mental health "detectives." Although they obtain a lot of important information about a patient during the extended initial examination, this information is rarely complete. Thus, psychiatrists often seek the patient's permission to obtain medical records from other doctors involved in the patient's care, including prior psychiatrists, as well as records from any psychiatric hospitalizations. This information can be critical for diagnosis and treatment, so patients are strongly encouraged to give their psychiatrists permission to obtain these records. The more the psychiatrist knows about the patient, the better it is for everyone involved. Additionally, psychiatric diagnosis, like all medical diagnosis, is an ongoing endeavor, and patients can expect to have aspects of their history reviewed again at subsequent visits.

After the initial examination, patients can usually expect to have follow-up appointments. The timing of these visits can range from days to weeks to a month or more after the initial appointment, depending on the psychiatrist's judgment about the severity of the disorder and the need for rapid and repeated intervention. Subsequent visits will also range in duration, depending on the need for further diagnostic evaluation and the nature of the treatments being used. Typical follow-up visits last from 15 minutes to an hour. Shorter visits are usually associated with medication management where the focus is on how the patient is doing on a given medication, on side effects of the treatment, and on the possible need for changes in treatment. Longer visits can include additional diagnostic discussions as well as the use of specific forms of talk therapy. Some psychiatrists focus their practice on the medical aspects of mental disorders, including the use of medications. These psychiatrists often refer patients to psychologists or social workers for their expertise in psychotherapy or in interventions that help patients with the social aspects of their dysfunction (e.g., job or marital problems). Other psychiatrists prefer to incorporate psychotherapy into their own management, and visits to these psychiatrists are typically longer in duration. One of the great fallacies of managed health care in the United States is the emphasis that third-party payers (health care insurance companies) put on separating medical and psychological management, using psychiatrists only for the medical portion of treatment. In our opinion, this is extremely unwise because complete psychiatric care always involves both medical and social/psychological interventions.

Splitting these functions among providers can be done effectively, but great care has to be used to prevent problems with miscommunication. The division of effort is arbitrary at best. This will be discussed in greater depth later in the book.

Since psychiatric disorders are usually long-term problems, they often fluctuate over time, with periods of improvement punctuated by distinct periods of illness that can vary in severity. In some cases, the psychiatric disorder itself is chronic, meaning that it is likely to be present more or less continuously for very long periods of time (even for life). Thus, it is important for patients to understand that, once they are diagnosed, their involvement with a psychiatrist is likely to be a long-term venture, although the frequency of visits can vary widely depending on the state and severity of dysfunction. Another important aspect for patients to understand is that at the present time there are *no cures* for psychiatric disorders. At best, these illnesses are managed over time, and significant improvement in symptoms is the norm. Again, this aspect of psychiatry is no different from the rest of medicine. Common illnesses like hypertension (high blood pressure), diabetes, and epilepsy are chronic problems that are not cured either. They, like psychiatric disorders, are managed by a knowledgeable physician.

The Importance of Diagnosis

Earlier in this book, we emphasized the importance of psychiatric diagnoses. In a "truth in advertising" mode, we reiterate here that this emphasis strongly reflects our own biases about psychiatry. We come from a department of psychiatry that is deeply rooted in a "medical model" approach to the field. This means that we believe strongly that the study and treatment of psychiatric disorders should be approached using the same methods employed for other medical conditions. We believe that accurate diagnosis provides the psychiatrist with important information about the expected course of the disorder and with critical guidance in making decisions about treatment, just as it does in the rest of medicine. But a medical model approach does not imply that medications and biologic treatments like ECT are the best (or only) treatments for psychiatric disorders. In some cases, psychotherapy alone may be the best option. In most cases, a combination of approaches that emphasizes appropriate medication use along with appropriate talk therapy and social interventions is critical for achieving optimal outcomes. We stress the importance of this integrated approach later in the book.

Why is diagnosis so important? It enables a psychiatrist to talk effectively with patients, their families, and other physicians about the nature of the disorder, the treatments that are most likely to be beneficial, and the expectations going forward, including the expected patient response to certain treatments and the likely short- and long-term course of the disorder. In effect, a valid diagnosis is a prediction about the future, based on extensive medical literature and clinical experience about the course and treatment response of a given disorder. In our opinion, all treatment recommendations should be based on the diagnosis. For example, a patient with major depression is unlikely to experience significant improvement in mood from a Valium-type medication prescribed for anxiety. Similarly, a patient with schizophrenia is unlikely to benefit from antidepressant medication alone, but will need antipsychotic medication as well. Without accurate diagnosis, communication, prediction about outcome, and effective treatment are extremely difficult and haphazard. A disturbing trend in all of medicine is the tendency for some doctors to focus on just treating symptoms. Such an approach is likely to produce only short-term benefits and is more likely to be associated with the use of multiple, sometimes inappropriate medications (called "polypharmacy" in medical jargon). Polypharmacy often results in significant side effects, adverse medication interactions, and poor overall response in part because of side effects. As we discuss later, there are no perfect treatments—all have side effects. The choice of a particular treatment is based on the probability of positive response and the probability that a patient will tolerate the treatment. This analysis is called the "risk-benefit ratio" and is a standard for all medical practice.

Psychiatric Hospitalization

In general, psychiatric hospitalization is reserved for patients with very severe symptoms, usually involving some form of dangerousness to self or others. Dangerousness to self includes suicidal ideas, intent, or behavior, or profound self-neglect such that the patient does not or cannot take care of the basic needs of life, such as eating, drinking, and finding shelter. Psychiatric disorder usually lies at the root of these symptoms, and hospitalization is aimed at protecting the patient until the disorder is under better control. Dangerousness to others is typically manifested by outwardly directed acts of violence or explicit threats toward others. To the extent that these violent symptoms result from an underlying psychiatric disorder, hospitalization can be beneficial in protecting the patient and others. In some cases, however, it is not clear whether a psychiatric disorder is causing a given violent behavior, because violence itself does not necessarily imply the presence of a psychiatric illness, or even whether hospitalization is the right course for those whose psychiatric condition tends by its very nature to be violent (e.g., antisocial personality disorder). These distinctions can be very difficult to make, but at the very least, the determination of whether a violent individual should be in a psychiatric hospital must begin with psychiatric diagnosis.

In the great majority of cases, psychiatrists and their patients agree when there is a need for hospitalization: Patients are admitted "voluntarily" to the hospital and in effect "sign themselves in," as described in popular jargon. At times, however, a psychiatric disorder may be so severe that the patient lacks sufficient insight or judgment to cooperate with protection and treatment. In those cases, the patient may be detained in the hospital involuntarily. The initial period of involuntary hospitalization is defined by the local legal jurisdiction. In our region, this is 96 hours. Following this initial period of evaluation, the psychiatrist must petition the local court for longer detention that can range from weeks to months. Recurring judicial review is required for longer periods of involuntary hospitalization. This is an example of an appropriate interaction between the legal system and the medical system in order to decide on the balance between a patient's need for treatment and a patient's right to decide freely about the need for treatment. Contrary to popular opinion, family or friends cannot simply "sign a patient in" unless they are the patient's duly appointed legal guardian. Involuntary hospitalization is a complex medical-legal decision process. Furthermore, involuntary hospitalization does not mean that a patient is "incompetent." Incompetency is a complex legal (not medical) decision. Psychiatrists can participate in the process of having an individual declared legally incompetent by providing information about psychiatric function and mental status, but the ultimate decision is made by the legal system.

Following psychiatric hospitalization, patients can expect to resume outpatient care on a regular basis, usually within the first week after discharge from the hospital. Sometimes, a patient participates in a day hospital program (called a "partial hospital program" in some locales) for several weeks in order to continue treatment in a setting that is less intensive than an inpatient hospital setting but more intensive than follow-up in an outpatient office or clinic. Outpatient visits are much like the follow-up visits described earlier and focus on symptoms, continued re-evaluation of diagnosis, and treatment. Patients are often advised to return to normal activities as soon as possible, because such activities (at work, home, or school) can be extremely important in diminishing the consequences and stigma of illness.

Preventing the Complications of Psychiatric Disorders

Perhaps one of the most important contributions psychiatrists make is to prevent or minimize the complications of psychiatric disorders. Of these complications, suicide is usually the most devastating. It is estimated that 30,000 or more people commit suicide each year in the United States, with another 650,000 people seeking treatment in an emergency room for suicide attempts. To put these numbers in perspective, suicide accounts for about 1% of all deaths and a suicide occurs about once every 20 minutes or less in the United States. In terms of frequency, suicides outnumber homicides by 3 to 2. It is estimated that over 90% of individuals who commit suicide have a major psychiatric disorder. We believe this estimate is low, representing an underestimation resulting from misdiagnosis or incomplete information. Thus, completed suicide almost always reflects a psychiatric problem. Other characteristics associated with completed suicide include gender (men commit suicide more often than women, although women attempt suicide more often than men), age (older individuals are at higher risk), family history of suicide, acute intoxication, adverse life circumstances (e.g., living alone, job loss, and divorce, particularly among alcoholics), and prior history of suicide attempts. Psychiatrists must weigh all of these variables in assessing risk. The good news is that completed suicide is a rare event, and thus the laws of probability are on the side of prevention. The bad news is that almost all psychiatrists have to deal with a patient's suicide at some point in their career; here, even one death is one too many.

As we've discussed previously, violence is another complication of some psychiatric disorders. Fortunately, violent acts by individuals with these disorders are, like completed suicide, rare events. The psychiatrist's responsibility in preventing violence is focused on determining whether a psychiatric disorder plays a role in causing the violence. But again, with some psychiatric disorders that are associated with potential for violence by their very nature, it is unclear what role psychiatrists should actually play in prevention. In the case of antisocial personality disorder, for example, the legal system and not the medical system is often the more appropriate venue to handle violent behavior.

Other complications of psychiatric disorders include problems at home, school, and work. Sadly, many of these complications are misunderstood by both the lay public and some psychiatrists as being the "cause" of a psychiatric problem. For example, a common misstatement is that a patient "got depressed because he got divorced." In many of these cases, a careful history reveals that the individual was depressed long before the divorce occurred, and in fact, the depression was one of the major causes of marital discord. Depressed individuals can be very difficult to live with. They are sad, irritable at times, unenthusiastic, pessimistic, and disinterested in sex—a bad combination for a successful relationship. With effective treatment, many, if not all, of these characteristics abate. Similarly, major psychiatric disorders are often associated with some form of cognitive dysfunction, ranging from problems with the ability to focus one's thinking (concentration) to memory defects. Cognitive and motivational problems make it hard for patients to function and can lead to job loss and school dropout. Discussion about these complications and efforts to prevent them are major components of good psychiatric care. Because patients with psychiatric disorders can have altered thinking and perception and are prone to poor or impulsive judgment, psychiatrists usually advise them to defer major life decisions until their disorder is under better control.

Another set of complications is becoming increasingly recognized and may rival suicide and violence in terms of impact on health and survival. These complications have to do with adverse interactions between psychiatric and other medical disorders. As discussed elsewhere, having a serious medical disorder increases risk for certain psychiatric disorders. It is now clear, however, that having a psychiatric disorder, particularly major depression, has adverse effects on the outcome of coexistent medical conditions. This has been studied in detail in several medical illnesses, including heart disease (heart attacks and heart failure), diabetes, and cancer. Compared to nondepressed patients, individuals who have these serious illnesses along with depression are much more likely to have a worse outcome of their medical disorder, including premature death. The standard explanation for this phenomenon is that depressed patients don't take good care of themselves and this puts them at greater risk. While no doubt this can be a factor, recent studies indicate that the altered biology accompanying depression (e.g., lower heart rate variability) is also likely to play a role. In several medical disorders, treating the underlying depression can improve the outcome of the medical disorder. This is clearest in diabetes, but it may also be the case in heart disease and cancer. In these cases, the psychiatrist's expertise complements the care being given by internists, cardiologists, and oncologists. In all of these situations, the psychiatrist's medical background comes into play in determining the presence of a psychiatric disorder and in implementing appropriate management.

Some psychiatric disorders also are associated with increased risks of developing certain medical disorders and of lower life expectancy. This is clearly the case in schizophrenia in which the disorder is associated with greater risks of diabetes (twofold increase), cardiovascular disease (twofold increase), and sudden death (threefold increase). The causes of sudden death are not always certain, but often involve heart problems, such as severely irregular heart rhythms and heart attacks. Factors contributing to these adverse associations are complex, but include increased body weight (about 40% of people with schizophrenia are obese) and cigarette use (about 80% smoke). The default "cause" for the high prevalence of obesity and smoking in people with schizophrenia traditionally has been thought to be the restricted lifestyle that results from having a psychotic disorder, but the situation is now known to be more complex. For example, one of the genes linked to schizophrenia codes for a protein that allows nicotine to work in the brain (a nicotine "receptor"); thus the association of schizophrenia with smoking may have to do with the basic biology of the illness and not simply with lifestyle. In other cases, the use of nicotine may be an attempt on the part of the patient to "self-medicate" to help correct problems with concentration and thinking. Additionally, some of the treatments for schizophrenia, particularly many current antipsychotic medications, cause weight gain (obesity). This weight gain results in problems with sugar metabolism (leading to diabetes) and altered cholesterol metabolism. This "metabolic syndrome" can result in markedly increased risk of cardiac dysfunction. These various risk factors and complications contribute to recent observations indicating that patients with schizophrenia die about 20 or more years earlier than would otherwise be expected. Premature death of this magnitude ranks schizophrenia among the major "killers" (i.e., illnesses associated with early death) known in the United States and would likely result in a huge public outcry if it occurred in other, less stigmatized, segments of the population. For patients with severe mental disorders, psychiatrists are often their primary (or only) link to medical care. Here again, the medical background of psychiatrists is critical for early recognition of medical and metabolic complications and for serving as the conduit for appropriate care.

Take-Home Messages

- Psychiatrists are medical doctors who specialize in mental disorders. In the mental health care delivery system, they are the only professionals with medical training and are thus in the best position to determine the role that medical and neurological disorders play in influencing psychiatric symptoms and treatment.

- A psychiatric interview is a specialized form of medical examination that focuses on symptoms involving thinking, emotion, and motivation. After the initial interview, typical visits with a

psychiatrist range from 15 minutes to an hour in duration.
Follow-up appointments occur at variable intervals from more than
once a week to several months or longer.

- Psychiatric disorders often start early in life, during adolescence and
young adulthood. They are also often chronic problems, like
diabetes, hypertension, and arthritis. Therefore, ongoing psychiatric
care is likely to be a long-term venture. Psychiatrists cannot cure
mental disorders, but improvement in symptoms and function is the
norm with effective treatment. There is no one form of treatment
that is best for all patients. Effective treatment is best designed on an
individual-to-individual basis.

- Psychiatric hospitalization can play an important role in managing
complex psychiatric disorders. Hospitalization is largely directed at
diminishing risks to patients and others.

- In addition to diagnosing and treating mental disorders, psychiatrists
focus on preventing the complications of these disorders. Suicide is a
major, if still rare, complication of serious psychiatric illnesses. Other
complications include violence (also rare) and problems in function
at home, work, and school (common). Having a major psychiatric
disorder has a negative impact on overall health status and results in
a worse outcome for a number of general medical conditions.

···*five*···

Why Are Psychiatric Disorders
So Common?

Studies examining the frequency of psychiatric disorders in various populations are done by epidemiologists. These are scientists who investigate patterns of illnesses, as well as their causes and prevention. They play key roles in describing epidemics and in identifying factors associated with the spread of a disease in a population. Ideally, they would like to study an entire population, such as the entire US population or the entire population of New York City. However, that is usually impossible (due to the economic costs and logistical challenges associated with such a massive research undertaking), so epidemiological studies rely on obtaining representative "random samples" of the people of interest. Based on these random samples, epidemiologists use statistics to estimate the frequency of an illness in a large population (called the "prevalence" of the disorder) and the percent of the population that develops the illness over a defined period of time (called the "incidence" of the disorder). Admittedly, this is a crude description of the science of epidemiology. Nonetheless, for our discussion, these definitions will suffice.

How Common Are Psychiatric Disorders?

There have been several studies examining the frequency of psychiatric disorders in US populations. Examples include the Midtown Manhattan Study, which was conducted in the 1950s, and the Epidemiological Catchment Area (ECA) Study, which was conducted in the 1980s. More recent studies include the National Comorbidity Study (NCS), the National Comorbidity Study-Replication (NCS-R), and the National Epidemiologic Survey on Alcohol and Related Conditions (NESARC), among others. These large studies have provided important insights into the nature of psychiatric disorders in the United States. As we noted in Chapter 1, the data from the NCS and NCS-R obtained from 1990 to 1992 and 2001 to 2003, respectively, indicate that the prevalence of psychiatric disorders in the adult US population (ages 18–54 years) is estimated to be about 30% (i.e., about one in three persons had a diagnosable psychiatric disorder during those periods). Based on other data, the prevalence may approach 50% when considered from a lifetime perspective (i.e., one-half of the US population is likely to have a psychiatric disorder at some point in their lives). Those are staggering figures and are a strong indicator that almost every person in the United States has some contact, knowingly or not, with persons with mental illness. When we consider the complexity of the brain systems that may be involved in various psychiatric disorders, these figures may make sense. As mentioned in Chapter 2, our brain motivation and reward systems are critical for our survival. However, these systems can be easily hijacked by drugs of abuse; this likely contributes to the prevalence of the various substance abuse disorders. Similarly, our brains' emotional systems are critical for how we function and survive. For example, some degree of anxiety can be healthy and can help to motivate us to protect ourselves against an obvious threat. But the systems governing anxiety and fear are highly regulated and can be turned on and off by a variety of stimuli, both appropriately and inappropriately. It is not too much of a stretch of the imagination to see that perturbation or overuse of these systems can interfere with our everyday functions (e.g., too much anxiety can be crippling). The same may be true for brain systems involved with mood and perceptions.

You'll recall that some good news/bad news scenarios came out of NCS and NCS-R. The good news indicated that the prevalence of mental illness in the US adult population did not increase over the 1990s and that treatment for mental disorders increased over that time from about 12% of the population to 20%. The bad news was that, despite the increase in treatment, almost two out of three patients with a psychiatric diagnosis did *not* receive treatment. Additionally, about half of the patients treated for a mental disorder actually did *not* have a diagnosable mental disorder, possibly reflecting the tendency of some physicians to treat symptoms and not disorders. For example, a person may report feeling sad to a primary care doctor and then be prescribed an antidepressant. However, another doctor, inquiring a little more deeply, may find that this person does not meet diagnostic criteria for a clinical depression and thus probably does not require pharmacologic treatment. As noted earlier, sadness does not equal depression. Sadness without other symptoms suggestive of depression may be a healthy and realistic response to a situation. With a little bit of support and time, the sadness is likely to resolve.

The results from NCS-R are consistent with other studies. For example, a recent survey by the World Health Organization (WHO) indicated that about 25% of the US population has a psychiatric disorder, but that only about 15% of these people actually get treatment. The perverse "good news" in the WHO study is that those who were defined as "seriously ill" had about a one in two chance of getting treatment. That is, if you are really sick, you have a higher likelihood of getting treatment than if you are more mildly ill; unfortunately, a 50% chance of getting treatment means that a lot of seriously ill individuals are not getting the care they need. Taken together, these are sobering data and indicate that psychiatric disorders are very common but poorly understood and very poorly treated in the US health care delivery system.

Are Psychiatric Disorders Over- or Underdiagnosed?

It is extremely difficult to know whether psychiatric disorders are over- or underdiagnosed. Based on the treatment data from the major epidemiological studies just outlined, psychiatric disorders in the community appear to be undertreated. From the perspective of medical practice, it would be logical to attribute this finding to underdiagnosis, particularly in primary care settings where training in psychiatry is limited and physicians are strapped for time. However, in the larger context of the society in which we live, the stigma of having a mental illness and the socioeconomic and cultural disparities in health care delivery also play a role. Based on NCS-R, there are clear social and economic variables that contribute to undertreatment, particularly disparities based on race and income level: If you come from an impoverished minority group, your chances of getting treatment for a psychiatric disorder are markedly diminished. Lack of knowledge about mental disorders, particularly among less educated and poorer people, is also likely to be a significant issue. Understanding how economic, educational, and cultural barriers result in reluctance to seek, or impede access to, treatment is important. In addition to these factors, certain psychiatric disorders are associated with poor insight into the need for treatment and even with fear of the health care system.

There is, on the other hand, some concern in our society that some psychiatric disorders are either on the rise or are being diagnosed at greater rates. This seems particularly true of disorders that occur at the extremes of age.

For example, in the United States, there is an increase in the number of people diagnosed with Alzheimer's disease. Dementing illnesses such as Alzheimer's disease clearly occur more frequently in elderly populations, and the US population is aging; therefore, the increase is expected. However, should we expect the rate at which childhood disorders such as autism are diagnosed to increase? Autism used to be considered rare, but now most of us have friends or relatives who are dealing with the disorder. Has there been a recent increase in autism and related disorders, or has recognition of autism improved? Again, this is a difficult question to answer confidently. Popular belief suggests that the prevalence of autism is increasing, but this may simply reflect two diagnostic trends: (1) an increased alertness on the part of clinicians, as well as parents and teachers, to childhood difficulties in social activities and school performance; and (2) a shift in diagnosis away from mental retardation syndromes toward autism. Some data suggest that the frequency of mental retardation diagnoses has diminished over the same time period that autism has appeared to increase—a diagnostic shift, so to speak.

Certain mood disorders, including major depression and perhaps bipolar disorder, may be increasing among children and adolescents. As a result, children are being treated with more psychiatric medications than they were in the past, including stimulants (e.g., Ritalin [methylphenidate] and amphetamine salts such as Adderall), antipsychotics (e.g., Risperdal [risperidone]), antidepressants (e.g., Prozac [fluoxetine]), and mood stabilizers (e.g., lithium). This represents an increase in both the number of children being treated and the number of powerful psychiatric medications being used. While there are good clinical data indicating that stimulants can be effective for treating attention deficit hyperactivity disorder (ADHD), the effectiveness of the other medications in major mood disorders in children is less certain.

If serious psychiatric illnesses are substantially increasing in our young, as experts in child psychiatry in particular believe, the reasons are likely to reflect changes in the environment rather than in genetics, given the relatively short time period over which the apparent increases have occurred. The nature of the responsible environmental changes are presently unclear, but could include problems that adversely affect a child's prenatal and postnatal development, such as maternal infection during pregnancy, early postnatal stress, abuse and neglect, poor diet, toxin exposure, and others. Investigating these possibilities, as for any environmental variables that may contribute to any complex illness, is extremely difficult from a scientific perspective. The studies needed to sort out these variables are time-consuming, require large population samples, and call for longer-term follow-up of individuals at risk with appropriate control groups. Thus, we have to be careful about jumping to premature conclusions about any contributing factors (e.g., vaccinations, television, day care, etc.), because premature conclusions can lead to interventions that do more harm than good. The "law of unintended consequences" comes readily to mind.

Another factor that could contribute to overdiagnosis is the identification of psychiatric disorders by primary care physicians. For instance, as mentioned earlier, a busy internist may diagnose as "depressed" a patient who says that she is sad because of relationship problems. If the physician had time for further discussion, it may become apparent that the patient is having a normal reaction to breaking up with a boyfriend and that her sleep, appetite, concentration, and interest in life—cardinal symptoms of major depression—are all fine. In other words, it is sometimes easy to overreact to such words as "depressed" or "sad" and to diagnose a clinical depression even when the low mood is a natural and normal reaction to an acute situation and requires no specific intervention.

The Interaction of Genes and Environment

Despite concern about possible overdiagnosis, sound epidemiological data indicate that psychiatric disorders are common. With this in mind, we return now to the question at hand: *Why* are psychiatric disorders so common? The answer is extremely complex, and one in which all the pieces of the puzzle are not completely understood at this time. It is likely, however, that the answer will come in part from a better understanding of human genetics and of the interaction between our genes and our environment in making us who we are.

Psychiatric disorders fall into a broad class of illnesses that geneticists refer to as "complexly inherited." This phrase means that a disorder results from interactions between a combination of multiple genes and their environment. Complexly inherited disorders represent most of the common maladies in medicine (e.g., diabetes, high blood pressure, obesity, and many cancers). Importantly, complex disorders, psychiatric disorders included, are *not* single-gene illnesses, meaning that no one gene defect causes them. This is different from "single-gene disorders" such as the one we described in Chapter 2—Huntington's disease, a major neuropsychiatric illness characterized by dementia and peculiar, jerky, uncontrollable movements called "chorea." In a "dominantly" inherited disorder like Huntington's disease, inheriting one abnormal gene from either parent is sufficient to get the illness. If you get the gene, you get the illness. But with common psychiatric disorders, single genes do not cause illness. A person inherits multiple genes that increase the relative "risk" for a given disorder. It is not known how many genes are required, but it is likely to be a lot—more than 10, maybe more than 100. Each gene, by itself, contributes very little to the overall risk. Thus, to get one of these disorders, a person may inherit many genes associated with the disorder or inherit a few genes that interact with something else. That something else is the environment.

In any discussion of human genetics, it is important to understand that the purpose of our genes is not to cause illness or dysfunction. Rather, genes are better thought of as biological tools that help humans to adapt and evolve— they are the agents that allow us to survive various challenges and the agents that have allowed us to evolve to our current state. The most important thing that humans adapt to is their specific environment. Events in the environment are detected by various sensors in our bodies. When these sensors are stimulated, they send signals to various tissues and cells. These signals can tell the pancreas to secrete more or less insulin, the adrenal gland to secrete more or less of the stress hormone cortisol, and so on. Eventually these signals can influence the genes located in the nuclei of our cells. Depending on the signal and the cell type, the genes may respond by causing changes in those cells or causing those cells to produce chemicals that influence other cells.

All of our cells, with the exception of eggs and sperm, contain exactly the same sets of genes, but cells differ with regard to which genes are turned on ("expressed") at any given time. Thus, a kidney cell has the same genes as a muscle cell and a nerve cell. The local environment of the cell within the body, as determined in part by the larger external environment of the individual, helps to determine which genes are expressed and where they are expressed. For example, chemicals that bathe a cell in the brain, including neurotransmitters, hormones, and growth factors, determine what genes are turned on in that nerve cell and how that nerve cell functions. Similarly, the connections of the nerve cell to other nerve cells helps to determine which proteins are expressed by the cell and which cells that nerve cell makes connections with. This is a dynamic situation that can change over the lifetime of the cell, depending on the types of activity and influences that the nerve cell experiences. Importantly, the local chemical and connectivity environment of the cell regulates the fact that the cell is a nerve cell and not a kidney or muscle cell. Understanding how the cellular milieu influences and directs gene expression is a very hot topic these days in cell biology and lies at the heart of efforts to regulate what are called "stem cells," the cells in our bodies that have the potential to become any other cell depending on what instructions they receive.

Regulation of gene expression occurs by a variety of mechanisms, but one process that may be important in brain function is called "epigenetics." The term (literally meaning "upon genetics") refers to changes that occur in genes or gene-associated proteins as a result of chemical modifiers of those genes/proteins. These chemical modifiers regulate whether a gene is turned on or not; they do not change the actual material, DNA (deoxyribonucleic acid), that make up the genes themselves. Epigenetic changes include chemical "tags" on DNA or on the proteins (histones) that help to package the genes. Chemically changing these tags, for example by adding or removing a methyl or acetyl group, can lead to changes in the amount of the "tagged" DNA that is translated into specific proteins. In turn, these specific proteins influence cell function. Epigenetic changes are not the same as "mutations," which change DNA composition and can result in altered protein structure and function.

Epigenetic changes involving certain cells in the brain are critical for determining how we learn and remember new information (or more specifically how our nerve cells learn and remember). Again, epigenetic changes do not reflect actual physical changes in genes; instead, they are produced by a kind of chemical tagging of genes that influences whether the tagged genes are turned on or turned off. Interestingly, epigenetic tags can be passed on to our children. Thus, children can carry reminders of what their parents experienced. For example, studies in rodents demonstrate that pups carry epigenetic reminders of the type of mothering they received after birth or of maternal exposure to alcohol or other drugs before they (the offspring) were born. In turn, these changes can be passed on to their offspring and influence how the next generation develops. Recent data from Michael Meaney's laboratory in Montreal indicate that some epigenetic changes in "stress receptors" observed in the brains of maltreated rats are also found in the brains of human suicide victims who were also victims of childhood abuse.

Overall, the process of regulating gene expression helps us adapt to our environments—whether stressful or pleasant. However, our genes are not "geniuses," so to speak, and what is adaptive in one environment may not be adaptive in another. For example, having a heightened fear response may help you survive in a jungle or inner city, but it may lead you to be overly fearful and anxious in a nonthreatening social interaction. The important point is that, with regard to common illnesses, humans inherit probabilities (or "liabilities") of developing an illness. The higher the genetic liability, the easier it is for environmental events to interact with the genetic risks and lead to illness. Genetic probabilities are usually not large enough to guarantee that a person will develop a specific psychiatric illness, but when they are combined with the "wrong" environment, disorders can occur. Single-gene disorders such as Huntington's disease are the rare disorders where the probability of getting the disorder is 100% when one inherits the gene for the disease. By contrast, the development of common disorders involves the combination of genetic predisposition, as determined by the summation of a large number of genes, together with environmental factors that influence some of these genes.

We presently know very little about what factors in the environment increase the risk of various disorders, but this is an important area of current research. One concern, however, is that being raised in a harsh environment, perhaps one with lots of stress and childhood abuse, may have long-term consequences on genes that may be difficult to reverse. Our genes may want to adapt, but the environmental events that may occur during certain stages of development may make it harder for our genes to adapt in a positive manner. Thus, undoing the effects of a bad environment may be extremely difficult, depending on whether the adverse experiences occurred during critical periods of development. In some ways, the effects of a harsh environment may be less forgiving than our genes. On a positive note, many people exposed to even the harshest of environments are quite resilient and manage to overcome or to be relatively unscathed by the experience. What makes some people so resilient and others so vulnerable is unknown and represents an area that we need to understand, for here may lie some of the keys to better treatments for psychiatric disorders.

To put this discussion into a psychiatric perspective, we will use the devastating psychotic illness, schizophrenia, as an example. In the general population, schizophrenia occurs in about 1 in 100 people (1% of the population). Having a parent or a sibling with the disorder increases the occurrence to about 15 in 100 people (15%). When both parents have schizophrenia, about half (50%) of the children have the disorder. Thus, the more genetic "whammy" one inherits, the higher the probability of getting the disorder. Another way to study this is to find out what happens to twins. Identical twins (called "monozygotic" or one-egg twins) have identical genes, whereas fraternal ("dizygotic") twins share only 50% of their genes. In single-gene disorders (e.g., Huntington's disease), if one identical twin gets a disorder, the other twin will get the disorder, assuming that the gene has complete (100%) "penetrance" (i.e., the gene is always completely expressed). In schizophrenia, studies have shown that the sibling of an identical twin with schizophrenia has about a 50% chance of getting the disorder. This important result tells us that genes cannot be the sole determinants of schizophrenia, although there is clearly a significant genetic risk involved. This means that environmental variables must contribute. Several environmental risk factors for schizophrenia have been identified, including complications at birth (e.g., low oxygen, premature birth, low birth weight) as well as prenatal exposure to certain infections, toxins (maternal alcohol abuse and lead exposure may be examples), or such other stressful conditions as malnutrition. Environmental stressors during early childhood development, including exposure to trauma, social isolation, and immigration, may be risk factors for the disorder as well. It also appears that abuse of certain drugs, such as marijuana, during late childhood and adolescence may increase the risk, especially when associated with particular genetic risks involving the gene for an enzyme called catechol-O-methyl-transferase (COMT), which affects the metabolism of key chemical transmitters in the brain.

There are some major "environmental" changes that may not be considered stressors but that may have potential to disrupt brain systems. For example, scientists are just now learning about the possible effects of dietary changes on our bodies. Over the last century or so, diet in western cultures has changed dramatically in terms of certain core nutrients (e.g., resulting in fewer essential omega-3-fatty acids), and some of these changes may play a significant role in heart disease, depression, and several other disorders. Similarly, we know little about the effects of obesity on our brain. Factors contributing to obesity include nutritional changes, decreased exercise, and increased time doing sedentary activities like watching television, riding in cars, and playing computer games. These "environmental" changes may lead to epigenetic changes that are passed on to future generations. Figuring out whether some of these "environmental" changes are influencing mental health, and, if so, which disorders and which environmental features, will be difficult and will require the expertise of multiple scientific disciplines.

In summary, everyone inherits some vulnerability to various common illnesses, including psychiatric disorders. This is simply part of the risk of being human. Our genes, however, do not always dictate whether a disorder will occur. Rather, our genes work in concert with the environment to determine who and what we become, as well as what illnesses we develop. Gene expression is very dynamic and always active, as indicated by the fact that we can learn and remember new things throughout our lives. Thus, even in the presence of certain genetic liabilities and adverse environments, there is still a reasonable chance that we will do okay in the long haul, at least for certain illnesses. One clear example comes from those studies we just cited of schizophrenia in identical twins, showing that when one twin is diagnosed with schizophrenia, the other twin has only a 50% chance of developing the illness despite the fact that they have identical genes. This implies a degree of human "plasticity," and as we'll discuss in more detail later, reflects one of the areas of great optimism for the field of psychiatry.

How Do Complex Genetics Translate into Common Disorders?

This is one of the major questions of modern genetics. One guess involves the idea that multiple paths (genetic, environmental, and neural) likely lead to psychiatric symptoms and disorders. For example, you can get an illness like schizophrenia because you have a particular genetic makeup that influences the function of specific neural circuits in your brain (e.g., the prefrontal cortex or the dopamine reward system). In a person with high genetic risk, environmental triggers may not need to be intense in order for the disorder to occur. Alternatively, you may have only a moderate genetic risk, but if really stressful things happen to you—or you make stressful things happen by taking certain drugs, for example—some of the brain systems underlying your thinking, emotion, and motivation could be disrupted and, in combination with the moderate genetic risk, result in your getting the disorder. Some people may be lucky and have very little genetic risk for certain disorders and, even in the face of a large environmental challenge, may still be protected.

A related idea is that psychiatric disorders are "heterogeneous" (i.e., they vary in how they manifest themselves). For example, schizophrenia is probably not a single disorder. Rather, it is more likely a family of illnesses with some similar features but also with subtle and not so subtle differences. Some people with schizophrenia have obvious persecutory (sometimes mistakenly called "paranoid") delusions: They believe, for example, that other people are trying to harm them. Others have noticeably illogical and incoherent thinking, with silly emotional responses. And a third group has severely impoverished thought, speech, and actions. All could be diagnosed as having "schizophrenia," but to even casual observers, there are clear differences among these people. Heterogeneity is likely to be even more pronounced for illnesses such as depression, as noted in Chapter 2. These differences in symptoms and clinical picture in psychiatric disorders (called "phenotypic heterogeneity" in genetic terminology) are a major challenge for the field of psychiatric genetics. To try to deal with this problem, some researchers are searching psychiatric disorders that run in families for core features that reflect the underlying brain dysfunction that causes illness. These features are called "endophenotypes" (a word that loosely translated means "internal characteristics"), and it is hoped that these endophenotypes have clearer genetic and neural underpinnings than the broad clinical syndromes described in DSM-IV. Examples of endophenotypes might include changes seen in brain imaging studies (e.g., changes in the size, shape, or function of the hippocampus) or specific difficulties with cognitive tasks involving attention and working memory.

Additionally, a great deal of work in genetics is trying to decipher the factors that contribute to human genetic variation. Although we have a lot of genetic material in our cells (more than 3 billion base pairs), we only have about 25,000 actual genes (some plants actually have more genes than we do), and only a percentage of these genes codes for proteins. Thus, the number of genes we have cannot account for all of our diversity. However, it is believed that there are close to 15 million places in our genetic material where one of the chemical components in our DNA can differ among humans (called "single nucleotide polymorphisms," or SNPs). This creates the opportunity for lots of variation among humans, and it is hoped that understanding what SNPs are and what they do will help us understand how we are so diverse, how illnesses occur, and why certain illnesses are so common.

Take-Home Messages

- Psychiatric disorders are very common. As many as one in two individuals may have a psychiatric disorder at some point during their lifetime. Overall, these disorders appear to be underdiagnosed in general medical settings.

- It is unclear whether the prevalence of childhood disorders is increasing in the population, but this is a concern given the frequency with which children are being treated with powerful psychiatric medications. Some disorders such as autism and related disorders do appear to be increasing, but the reasons are not certain.

- Psychiatric disorders are "complexly inherited." This means that they typically reflect the effects of many genes as well as the interaction of the environment with genes. Importantly, genetic inheritance alone does *not* dictate whether a psychiatric disorder will occur. Thus, if you have a psychiatric disorder, your children are at increased risk of having that psychiatric disorder as well, but the risk is far from absolute. The factors, such as resilience, that protect some individuals from developing psychiatric disorders, despite high genetic inheritance and harsh environment, are not fully understood but are now the focus of great research interest.

- Gene expression can change over time and is likely to be manipulated by changes in the environment. Environmental changes that occur during a person's prenatal and early postnatal life are becoming recognized as increasingly important factors in determining the onset of some psychiatric disorders.

- There appear to be multiple paths—genetic, environmental, and neural—that lead to psychiatric disorders. It is this complexity that likely helps drive, at least in part, the frequency of psychiatric disorders in the population. Thus, psychiatric disorders are in our genes . . . and in our environment . . . and in our brains.

···six···

What Do We Know about the Mechanisms Underlying Psychiatric Disorders?

The Holy Grail of psychiatric science is to understand the biological mechanisms underlying mental illnesses. It is hoped that once we are armed with this information, we will be able to devise new strategies that target the primary brain dysfunctions and that possibly prevent these complex and devastating disorders from occurring in the first place. Realistically, we are a long way from these goals. However, rapid advances in neuroimaging, neuroscience, and genetics over the latter part of the last century give us strong reasons for optimism. Some of the research techniques that are now routinely used in neurobiology laboratories on a daily basis were considered "Star Wars" science 15 or 20 years ago. For example, it is now common for scientists to use functional magnetic resonance imaging (fMRI) to examine changes in brain function associated with human cognition and emotion. Similarly, laboratory scientists now routinely can add specific genes (called "knock-in") or eliminate specific genes (called "knock-out") from specific regions of rodent brains to assess how those genes and their products influence nerve-cell function, behavior, and learning. In this chapter, we will discuss some of what scientists, as a result of these advances, are learning about the biology of psychiatric disorders. This is not meant to be a comprehensive discussion, but rather a sampling of the exciting findings that neuroscience and genetics research has generated in recent years.

In this discussion, we start from the simple position that the "human mind" is a product of the "human brain." Thus, when we talk about mechanisms, we are talking about "brain mechanisms." In a broad sense, your brain is you—how you think, feel, and experience the world around you, all qualities of the mind. While we don't pretend to understand for certain how the human brain produces the human mind, we believe strongly that understanding the intricacies of how the brain works will ultimately help us to understand how the mind, along with the psychiatric disorders that affect it, is generated from brain activity.

"Chemical Imbalance" Means "We Don't Know"

When patients ask their psychiatrists what is going on in their brains that causes their depression or hallucinations or other symptoms, they are asking very complex questions that are difficult to answer easily. Questions about how psychiatric medications work are similarly complex. Many psychiatrists answer simply that psychiatric disorders are "chemical imbalances" in the brain and that the medications correct these "imbalances." Significantly, we know a lot more about how psychiatric drugs affect important neurotransmitter systems in the brain than we know about how these disorders actually occur in the brain. Thus, psychiatrists are usually adept at explaining how medications affect neurotransmitters such as gamma-aminobutyric acid (GABA), dopamine, norepinephrine, or serotonin. This information is based on reasonable scientific studies. What is much less clear is whether the known drug actions have anything to do with the fundamental problems that lead to psychiatric dysfunction and disturbed thinking, emotion, and motivation. That is, medications can have very specific effects on very specific proteins in the brain or other body organs, but this does not necessarily imply that abnormal function of those proteins causes the disorder. Indeed, many of the remedies used in medicine involve the treatment of symptoms and not the underlying pathology. A clear example is the use of aspirin or acetaminophen (Tylenol) for treating fever. These agents work very well to lower fever, but they have nothing to do with the "cause" of the fever. Similarly, most treatments for pain are effective but have nothing to do with the cause of the pain. Likewise for many psychiatric medications: They may influence the symptoms of psychiatric illnesses, but it is likely that they do not directly address the core defects that actually cause the particular illness.

Thus, the "chemical imbalance" or "leaky membrane" explanation of psychiatric illness says more about how a medication is likely to influence various brain transmitters than about what is actually wrong with the brain that leads to the illness. The fact is that, from a neuroscientific perspective, we presently don't know the causes or mechanisms underlying any major psychiatric disorder. The good news, however, is that we do know a lot about how current psychiatric medications influence various brain systems, and this knowledge is informing the development of newer and even more effective treatments. In time, such knowledge may bring us closer to understanding the nature of the primary brain abnormalities that actually cause these illnesses, but right now, that understanding is elusive and in any case is hardly captured by the statement that an illness results from "a chemical imbalance." That is about as useful as saying that "something isn't quite right in the brain."

How the Brain Functions and Malfunctions: Current Science and Theory

All psychiatric disorders involve dysfunctions of the human brain. Contributing variables include our genetics and our environment, but the underlying mechanisms of the disorders involve brain abnormalities. At what level the dysfunction occurs is one of the major questions in the field. The human brain is a complex organ, and this complexity can make it difficult to study. Take, for example, the specialized nerve cells called "neurons." Roughly 100 billion in number, these cells do the primary work of the brain. Although there are differences among neurons in different regions of the brain, and although they have been given different names (e.g., pyramidal neurons, interneurons [of which there are many types], granule cells, stellate neurons, etc.) often based on their shape and function, neurons are all alike in some basic ways: They all send and receive chemical signals, and they all are electrically excitable. What seems to be critical for how neurons function is both their pattern of connections to other nerve cells and to other regions of the brain and the mechanisms by which those connections develop, are maintained, and influence the genes that are expressed in a specific neuron. Each neuron has something like 10,000 connections called "synapses." Adding to this complexity is the likelihood that there may be as many as 10 times more supporting cells in the brain (called "glia" or "glial cells") than neurons. But these glial cells provide much more than just structural support for neurons; glia are now recognized as key participants in brain energy balance and information processing. The brain is a very demanding beast when it comes to energy use; although it weighs only about 3 pounds, it requires about one-fourth of the output of the heart in order to sustain brain function. If you shut down heart function, even briefly, you shut down the brain. Additionally, there is enormous complexity in the way the various cells in the brain change with environmental input. Such changes are responsible for thinking, emotions, and motivation.

Psychiatrists vary widely in their approach to dealing with this complex organ. All psychiatrists have some training in neurology, so they understand how damage to the nervous system can alter sensory, motor, and cognitive function. Beyond this, there is some debate about how much clinical psychiatrists should actually know about neuroscience. Some psychiatrists treat the brain as the proverbial "black box." Information comes in, gets processed, and results in output in terms of behavior, thoughts, and mood. These psychiatrists are not particularly interested in knowing what goes on inside the brain; instead, they focus on observable outputs and on changing those outputs that are dysfunctional. Today, this "black box" view is probably held by a minority of psychiatrists, since advances in pharmacology and other treatments make this position much less tenable than it was 50 years ago. Other psychiatrists view the brain as a chemical or electrical organ and approach psychiatric problems from this perspective. This is, in effect, the approach some use in discussing drug treatment and has led to the overly simplistic "chemical imbalance" concept. Still other psychiatrists are those involved in brain research: They attempt to understand the critical interconnections within the nervous system and the ways in which those connections can be modified to influence behavior and thinking. Although this work is still a long way from having clinical applications and is therefore of little use to practicing psychiatrists now, it is the focus of a lot of today's leading neuroscience research and holds much promise for tomorrow's practitioners.

Numerous neuroscientists have attempted to develop better conceptual models about how the brain works relative to psychiatric disorders. These approaches, as exemplified by Joseph LeDoux in his book *Synaptic Self*, start with the idea that the brain is organized into parallel systems that serve specific and interacting functions. These systems allow us to process information simultaneously from both the external world (using our five senses) and our internal world and to generate various types of emotions, movement, thoughts, and behaviors. "Internal-world" processing systems include neural circuits that regulate wakefulness, vital bodily functions such as breathing, and other bodily activity (e.g., various hormonal processes). Additionally, our brains are equipped with a critical system that continuously monitors our internal bodily state relative to what is going on in the external world. Cognitive neuroscientists such as Marcus Raichle refer to this as a "default" system, so named because it is the default state to which our brains naturally relax when not doing other things. The areas of the brain involved in this continual monitoring are located deep within the neocortex and include highly connected midline regions (one area is called the cingulate cortex, and another is the precuneus). This default system uses a lot of energy, and interestingly, some of the earliest changes that occur in Alzheimer's disease involve these default-system brain regions; in fact, it may be the high activity and energy demands of these regions that render them so vulnerable to Alzheimer's disease.

Other brain systems allow us to focus our attention on specific things that we are thinking about, to set and monitor goals, and to use language both as input and output devices. But when we focus our attention on something, our brains must shift out of the default-processing state and into a state that engages parts of prefrontal cortex involved in "working memory." The contents of working memory are the items we are thinking about right now, such as keeping the previous sentences in mind as you read this sentence or remembering a phone number for a brief period of time. Working memory has limited capacity, so its contents must be refreshed and updated frequently in order to remain active in our conscious minds. These states of focused attention involve decreases in energy use in the default system and increases in blood flow and energy use in the brain regions required for the specific type of processing. There is considerable interest these days in understanding whether defects in shifting in and out of the default state may be important in some psychiatric disorders. Such defects may partly explain, for example, why patients with illnesses like depression, schizophrenia, or obsessive-compulsive disorder are so preoccupied with their internal world that they seem oblivious to things going on around them.

Our brains perform very complex activities that can range from processing simple perceptions to forming complex abstract thought, language, music, and mathematics. The systems that perform these sorts of tasks are actually fairly simple in their design and are built the way the nervous systems of other organisms and animals function. This point has been emphasized cogently by neuroscientist David Linden in his book, *The Accidental Mind*. Linden points out how complex human brain systems are layered upon more primitive systems and have evolved in a manner that has both expanded on the primitive functions seen in the brains of other animals and allowed for increased complexity. Understanding how this increased complexity actually occurs remains a major goal of current research, but it likely results from how the various regions of our brain are wired together and influence each other.

There are several key brain systems that seem to make up the human "mind." For now, it is important to understand that all of these systems are continuously processing and generating information. Sometimes we are aware consciously of what is going on, and sometimes this processing occurs outside of our conscious awareness. A major challenge for the brain is how to coordinate this activity across all of these systems and to produce a coherent picture of the self and the world. This is a very difficult task, one that computers have not been able to duplicate. In fact, our brains don't always do this coordination task very well either, and this may be one of the defects in processing that contributes to neuropsychiatric disorders. In some cases, a breakdown in information transfer between the various brain systems can lead to very peculiar behaviors and thoughts. For example, after suffering a stroke that affects the nondominant brain hemisphere, a person develops paralysis of the left arm. The nondominant hemisphere is the nonlanguage side of the brain; this is the right hemisphere in most people. What is peculiar about the people who experience these nondominant hemisphere strokes is that they also may lose the ability to recognize that their paralyzed arm is part of their own body. They may perform all kinds of complex behaviors but completely ignore the left side of their bodies (called "hemi-neglect," or "anosognosia" [literally, lack of awareness of a defect or disease]). For example, if they are asked to draw a clock, they may put numbers only on the right side of the clock. If asked to read the word *woman*, they may report seeing only the word *man*. You can imagine the kinds of problems this can create. Other peculiar disconnection syndromes include such states as "alexia without agraphia" (literally, deprived of words but not deprived of writing), in which the person can write but cannot read his or her own writing. This syndrome results from a defect in the ability to transfer information between the left and right cerebral hemispheres via a major connection pathway called the corpus callosum.

It doesn't take a lot of extrapolation to realize that aberrant or dysfunctional connections between neural systems could lead to other odd behaviors, including perhaps psychotic symptoms. For example, some patients with schizophrenia develop the false belief that a loved one has been replaced by an exact "double" (called "Capgras syndrome" after the individual who described such patients). Although we do not know what actual defect causes Capgras syndrome, cognitive neuroscientists such as V.S. Ramachandran suggest that these individuals have a disconnection between perceptual and emotional systems in the brain. Thus, when they see their loved one, they don't experience the appropriate and expected positive emotion, and their brains then make up a story to explain the lack of emotion (i.e., "this can't be my mother because I don't feel anything for her; the person must be an imposter").

The idea that such disconnection can occur is not much of a jump in logic from what we know about how our brains function normally. Even when working normally, our conscious brain may not be getting complete stories from its various subsystems. Under these circumstances, our conscious mind tends to "fill in the blanks" and make up stories to explain things. This is the basis for some amazing tricks of the mind, including our responses to Gestalt images of a complex or incomplete scene in which our mind actually "sees" lines or images that aren't really there. It is in fact quite amazing that our brains work as well as they do, given the enormous number of neurons, synapses, and systems that are operating all the time and the need for continuous coordination across these systems to produce coherent thinking and behavior. One of the current leading efforts in cognitive neuroscience is the attempt to use neuroimaging techniques to develop "connectivity" maps of our brains to understand in greater detail how brain regions are functionally interconnected and how those interconnections may go awry in various illnesses.

What Brain Systems Contribute to the Human Mind?

This brings us to a fundamental question: What is known about the neural systems underlying mental function? Again borrowing from Joseph LeDoux and his book *Synaptic Self*, we think about the mind in terms of the things it does— thinking, feeling, and motivating. In simplest terms, thinking or cognition is our ability to focus attention on a specific issue and to hold that idea or perception "online" (to use computer jargon) in our working memory— "to hold that thought," as it were. We are equipped with several important areas of the brain that help this process. LeDoux refers to these areas as "convergence zones" where information from our senses and higher-order systems are combined, allowing us to form high-level associations. That is, we are not bound by simply sensing the things around us and within us; we can also develop more complex, abstract thoughts that become part of the mix and lead to even more complex abstractions. An example of this property can be seen in our mathematical abilities. Initial, concrete conceptualizations (e.g., counting on our fingers) are driven by our senses, but we can later use these basic concepts to develop more abstract ways (e.g., the number line, two- and three-dimensional graphs, geometry, and algebra) to think about things. The areas in our brains that do this type of integration are highly connected with other areas of the brain, and it is this high degree of connectedness that probably allows the synthesis of information. We've already mentioned one critical area for bringing this processing to consciousness, and it is the so-called working-memory area of the brain, located, in part, in the upper (dorsal) outside (lateral) part of the prefrontal cortex (PFC). The dorsolateral PFC (and regions highly connected to the PFC) allows us to keep a certain number of items in consciousness, and this working-memory function is probably the closest thing in neuroscience to what we mean by a conscious "thinking" area of the brain. Again, human working memory has limited capacity; that is, only a certain number of items can be kept online for processing. For most of us, this is about seven items (the length of most local phone numbers), and the contents of working memory have to be refreshed regularly to keep those items in our consciousness.

One of the big evolutionary advances for humans was the marked increase in the size of our PFC. The enhancement of this brain region sets us apart from other species, including other primates. The human PFC has multiple subregions and allows us not only to think but also to plan, make predictions, draw inferences, and according to some neuropsychologists like Elkonon Goldberg, deal with ambiguity. According to Goldberg, the PFC is like a "chief executive officer" of the brain. Although it doesn't control all aspects of brain function, this region knows where to get critical bits of information from other regions and what part of the brain can best use that information. The PFC is also able to influence and regulate other regions of our brain by what is called "top-down processing." This means not only that humans process information from the "bottom up" (i.e., from our senses to our PFC), but also that our thoughts can influence our perceptions and actions. Defects in PFC function accompany many neuropsychiatric disorders, but these defects do not necessarily mean that the PFC itself is the site of brain damage. Rather, there are many pathways that lead to PFC dysfunction that then can result in complex thinking and behavioral abnormalities. That is, malfunction of the PFC can occur even when damage or misfiring is occurring in other regions of the brain, in part because the PFC is getting defective information. The susceptibility of the PFC to malfunction via multiple paths may be one of the reasons why psychiatric disorders are so common and why thinking abnormalities are common symptoms of these disorders.

Our minds also allow us to compute the value of things. These "valuation systems" are what neuroscientists call our emotions, and their presence reflects activity in specific neural circuits. There are debates about how many emotional systems actually exist in the human brain, but some anthropologists suggest that, across human cultures, there are six primary emotions—happiness, sadness, fear, anger, surprise, and disgust (some include a seventh, contempt). These emotional systems are built to process information very rapidly and outside of consciousness if necessary. They likely have played a big role in our survival as a species because they can lead to quick defensive actions. Fear is a great example. We can become quite afraid of something we don't even recognize, such as the unexpected movement of a shadow. We are startled and are ready to take protective actions well before our conscious brain recognizes that what we fear is just a plant moving in the breeze. Thus, the emotional systems are built to take charge when they are activated and can actually take over control from our thinking self. When under their singular influence, we often don't think very well at all.

Great advances are occurring in the research on the neural circuits underlying emotions. Most progress has been made in several labs, including LeDoux's, that have studied fear in animals and have highlighted the importance of a brain region called the amygdala. A walnut-shaped structure located deep in the temporal lobe of the brain, the amygdala receives input from sensory systems and has strong connections to hormonal systems and to regions of the PFC that are important for emotional processing. Interestingly, it is possible to activate the amygdala without going through the neocortex, providing an explanation for why conscious recognition of an emotion does not necessarily have to accompany an emotional experience, at least not immediately. When emotions and their attendant bodily changes (heart rate, sweating, breathing, etc.) reach consciousness in working memory, we experience what neuroscientist Antonio Damasio refers to as a "feeling."

Some scientists approach emotions from an evolutionary perspective that is based on the way animals normally behave. This approach makes intuitive sense, given that many of our brain systems are extensions of those found in the nervous systems of other animals. One of the leaders in this area is Jaak Panksepp. According to Panksepp, animals exhibit seven core emotions that might serve as "endophenotypes" for understanding some aspects of human psychiatric disorders. As you might recall from Chapter 5, the term *endophenotype* refers to characteristics arising from an organism's genetic and neural make-up that may signal the presence of more complex traits, such as psychiatric symptoms. An example of an "emotional endophenotype" might be an exaggerated startle response to innocuous stimuli. Such a startle response might predict abnormal fear/anxiety responses under other circumstances or even a disorder, such as generalized anxiety disorder. Some of the emotional systems that Panksepp identifies overlap with the emotions noted before, but there are interesting differences. Panksepp's seven emotional processes include "care" (maternal nurturance), "lust" (sexual drive), "play" (joyfulness), "fear" (freezing behavior when frightened), "rage" (anger), "panic" (separation distress), and "seeking" (motivation). These processes reflect activity in certain neural circuits and involve specific neurotransmitters and neurochemicals. Defects in or inappropriate use of these various systems could contribute to the emotional distress seen in psychiatric disorders, with different disorders exhibiting changes in different systems. For example, anxiety might be seen as dysfunction in the fear system, and low mood might result from perceived loss by the panic system. It is interesting that fear and panic are considered to be separate in this scheme; this may give some insight into differences in the emotional content of some disorders that result in anxiety with or without depression.

As described in Chapter 2, Panksepp's emotional process of "seeking" seems most akin to what is sometimes referred to as our "motivation system"— that is, the brain circuitry through which we set goals and take actions to reach those goals. This is an evolutionarily ancient system that is highly related to our brain's reward system. The details of how motivation and novelty/ reward-seeking function are being worked out in great detail at cellular and systems levels, and it appears that the neurotransmitter dopamine plays a major role. Activity ("firing") of neurons within the dopamine system in our midbrain appears to be regulated by whether a stimulus meets our expectation or not; release of dopamine onto other neurons when stimuli meet or exceed expectations helps bias those neurons to respond to specific inputs that are seen as rewarding. In effect, dopamine, acting in the PFC and other regions, tells neurons to pay attention and to filter out unimportant signals.

Many things motivate humans. Many motivators are basic life instincts, such as the drives to obtain food and sex. Because of the way the human brain is wired, we can also be motivated by our own thoughts ("top-down process-ing"). In fact, one thing that seems to separate humans from higher primates is the ability to be motivated by our own abstract ideas. As an example, neuro-scientist Read Montague, in his book *Why Choose This Book?,* notes how moti-vated some people are by religious or political ideas; as far as we know, humans may be the only species that is motivated by such abstract ideas and that will, at times, die for those ideas. As a function of its role in the motivation system, dopamine is particularly important in understanding the biology of drug and alcohol abuse. Most abused drugs can hijack the dopamine-related reward system. In effect, they alter dopamine release or uptake, and their presence can become a reward signal. Similarly, it appears that "normal" rewards such as food, sex, games, and thought can hijack the human reward system. Although it seems popular these days to discuss these rewards as "addictions," it is much less clear that food, sex, and other more "normative" rewards have the same impact on the dopamine system as abused drugs like cocaine, heroin, and alcohol. To us, it seems premature to include "food addiction" or "sex addic-tion" among addictive disorders, but it is an interesting issue that certainly warrants additional study. Other problems like chronic gambling and the seductiveness of our own thinking highlight the relative ease with which humans can focus their motivation. The difference between normal regula-tion of the reward system and abnormal manipulation of this system leading to addictive behaviors may have to do with the speed, amount, and pattern of stimulation. A burst of stimulation from snorting cocaine or injecting heroin has a very different effect on this system than the more gradual pleasure obtained from anticipating and eating a good meal.

How Are Diverse Brain Systems Coordinated?

It is a major challenge for our brain to coordinate activity across its various systems, especially when some of them, like the emotional systems, seem to do what they want to do when they want to do it. How the brain manages itself is an area of major interest in neuroscience and one that is becoming clearer as studies progress. As noted before, certain areas of our brain, particularly higher centers like the PFC, are well connected and receive input from multiple sources. These "convergence zones" (in LeDoux's phrase) integrate activity across other brain regions to help direct appropriate responses. One way that this integration is accomplished is through a process called "synaptic plastic-ity," which alters the strength of the connections between regions. Synapses are the highly specialized regions where neurons send and receive information from other neurons. Through the work of many neuroscientists, including the Nobel laureate Eric Kandel, it is now clear that synapses are highly complex and dynamic structures that are well equipped to change their functional activity and even their structure depending on input from other neurons and brain regions.

Related to this idea, it appears that our nervous systems are very skilled at detecting things that happen at the same time (called "coincidence detection" by neuroscientists). When two excitatory inputs to a neuron fire at or near the same time, the strength of these inputs is enhanced, leading to "long-term potentiation" (LTP; i.e., long-lasting enhancement of the synaptic connec-tions). Similarly, when two inputs are discoordinated in time, the strength of the connections is weakened, and this decrease may also be long lasting (called "long-term depression," or LTD). These important forms of synaptic adapt-ability are known as "Hebbian plasticity," after the psychologist Donald Hebb who first postulated that such changes could occur in the nervous system. In effect, Hebbian plasticity says that "neurons that fire together wire together." This process is a major step in the coordination of activity across systems in our brain.

Every region of the brain seems to be capable of Hebbian plasticity and thus capable of changing activity in response to changes in inputs. However, one region of the brain, the hippocampus, may be the grand master of Hebbian plasticity. The hippocampus plays a major role in learning and memory. It is also the place to which almost all other brain regions ultimately send information. The hippocampus, likely through synaptic plasticity, takes in this information and forms connections between the pieces of information being experienced. Information processing in the hippocampus is critical for short-term memory formation, allowing us to form connections among various thoughts, emotions, sensations, behaviors, space, and time. The hippocampus then feeds this information back to higher centers in the cortex for longer-term storage and additional processing. When information is recalled later, the hippocampus also appears to play a role, but in these cases, old information can be combined with new information, leading to yet newer memories that can be abstractions of the older memories. Again, coincidence in time and space are critical for how we tie pieces of information together in our brains.

As you might imagine, damage to the hippocampus can be devastating. Each side of the brain has a hippocampus; damage to both hippocampi leads to a syndrome in which individuals can take in new information but cannot hold onto it. Very shortly after experiencing something new, such individuals have no recollection of the new information. For example, a person with such damage can meet you and interact with you in meaningful ways. However, if you leave and then return 5 or 10 minutes later, the person will have no recollection of ever having met you. In effect, every experience is new. Interestingly, recall of information learned before the hippocampal injury is still reasonably intact, although even these older memories may be at least somewhat impaired. Alzheimer's disease is a common illness that involves gradual deterioration in this type of function. A person with this illness has increasing difficulty recalling recent events, but may have reasonable memory for events earlier in life.

How does our brain detect coincidences and coordinate activity across regions? For this discussion, it is important to understand that our brains use two major classes of neurotransmitters, the chemicals that transmit information between nerve cells. They are classified as "fast" or "slow," depending on the time course of their actions. Although there are exceptions to this classification and the descriptions are simplistic, fast transmitters are neurochemicals that are released from specialized endings of the neuron that is sending information and act on protein receptors on the surface of the nerve cell that is receiving information. Examples of fast neurotransmitters are glutamate and GABA. When these neurochemicals bind to their receptors, they open an ion channel that lets charged atoms (e.g., sodium, potassium, calcium, or chloride ions) enter or exit the receiving cell. The opening and closing of these ion channels occurs very quickly—on the order of milliseconds (one one-thousandth of a second)—and causes an immediate impact on the receiving cell. A certain type of glutamate receptor, the N-methyl-D-aspartate (NMDA) receptor, has the interesting property that its ion channel does not activate when neurons are at rest, even if glutamate binds to the receptor. Rather, activation of NMDA receptors requires that glutamate binds to the receptor *and* that the receiving neuron is already active by some other mechanism (e.g., by the actions of other excitatory receptors on the receiving cell). When both conditions are met, NMDA receptors become active and let calcium ions enter the receiving cell. By this type of mechanism, NMDA receptors function as "coincidence detectors," that is, they "sense" when glutamate is released from another cell at a time when their own cell is active. In turn, the calcium signal provided by NMDA receptors activates biochemical machinery in the receiving cell that can influence how effectively that cell's synapses function. These are the mechanisms that underlie synaptic plasticity, the process thought to be important for learning and memory. Additionally, changes in synaptic efficacy can last a long time (days or longer) and thus have the properties one would expect from a cellular memory mechanism.

NMDA receptors are key regulators of synaptic plasticity, but they are not the only receptors responsible for detecting coincident activity in the brain. A second class of neurotransmitters—the so-called slow transmitters—can play a significant role by altering the "tone" (or degree of activation) of nerve cells distributed throughout larger regions of the brain. These transmitters are "slow" because the receptors on which they act produce effects that develop relatively slowly and last for seconds, minutes, or even longer and influence the state of readiness of receiving cells. The slow transmitters have effects that are more broadly distributed throughout brain regions than the effects of the fast transmitters, giving these slow transmitters the ability to coordinate activity within and across regions. They also have longer-lived effects on the excitability of nerve cells, making the nerve cells and brain regions either more or less responsive to new inputs over longer periods of time. The slow transmitters are sometimes called "neuromodulators" and include chemicals like serotonin, dopamine, acetylcholine, and norepinephrine. These neurotransmitters are targets for many psychiatric medications and are thus thought to be involved in the biology of some psychiatric disorders. Additionally, even classical "fast" transmitters like glutamate and GABA can act on "slow receptors" to influence neural tone. The effects caused by the action of many types of slow transmitters determine the background level of activity against which the effects of the fast transmitters can be enhanced or diminished in local regions and across regions of the brain. Thus, these slow transmitters (and the medications that influence them) can be critical for determining how different regions of the brain work in concert, and they participate in processes like wakefulness and attention, which require coordinated brain activity.

There are some neurochemicals (e.g., growth factors, hormones, and peptide or small-protein neurotransmitters) that act on even slower time scales to coordinate growth of neurons and connections within the brain. Examples include nerve growth factor (NGF), brain-derived neurotrophic factor (BDNF), and others. Increasingly, these types of neuromodulators are being studied as possible targets for treatments in psychiatry and neurology.

What Are We Learning about the Brain in Psychiatric Disorders?

Psychiatric disorders are dysfunctions of the human mind. Thus, efforts to understand what goes wrong in these disorders focuses heavily on examining changes affecting the brain systems involved in thinking, emotions, and motivation. Although scientists do not yet fully understand the biology of any major psychiatric disorder, they are beginning to make significant progress in this area. In this section, we will briefly discuss as examples of this progress the results of recent investigations on three groups of disorders: substance abuse disorders, major depressive disorders, and schizophrenia.

Because of the ability of abused drugs to usurp brain reward pathways, we are probably closer to understanding the mechanisms underlying substance abuse disorders than we are to understanding those of any other psychiatric disorder. This field of study also greatly benefits from advances in human neuroimaging and animal research. Because of similarities between the rodent and human reward systems, it is possible to examine what happens when animals become "addicted" to specific drugs. A number of leading scientists, including Eric Nestler, Rob Malenka, and others, are making a great deal of progress in identifying short- and longer-term changes in the reward system as a function of chronic drug exposure. Importantly, the principles identified from these studies have dovetailed nicely with our increasing knowledge about synaptic plasticity and processes like long-term potentiation and long-term depression. In the short term, abused drugs have specific effects on dopamine and PFC systems, consistent with their known pharmacology. In the longer term, however, the brain adapts to the drugs, and there are lasting synaptic, cellular, and even structural changes that reflect how the brain adapts to repeated drug use. These long-term effects play a major role in determining why it is so difficult to reverse the effects of drug exposure. The studies examining these issues are identifying important cellular and genetic mechanisms involved in these adaptations and are nearing the point where new therapies for drug addiction may be possible.

Major depressions are another group of disorders in which significant research progress is being made. Human neuroimaging studies are playing a big role in these advances as well. In addition, there are now several useful animal models of depression that are based on chronic stress and "learned helplessness" in both rodents and nonhuman primates. In major depression, the circuitry linking the PFC (thinking), amygdala (emotions), reward system (motivation), and hippocampus (memory formation) is critically important. Investigators such as Wayne Drevets, Helen Mayberg, and others have identified a specific region in the brain, the "subgenual anterior cingulate cortex," as having abnormal metabolic and blood-flow activity during depression. This region is just below a bend ("genu") in the front part of the corpus callosum, the large bundle of fibers in the middle of the brain that plays a big role in connecting brain regions with one another, including the two cerebral hemispheres. Part of the PFC and a key player in a distributed system that appears to be critical for regulating mood, the subgenual anterior cingulate cortex shows structural changes reflecting a marked loss of certain glial cells in some individuals with depression. Interestingly, different treatments used for depression, including some forms of talk therapy, have differing and complementary effects on this circuitry. Similarly, studies by Yvette Sheline and other investigators have provided evidence that at least some patients with major depression also have structural changes (shrinkage) in the hippocampus and amygdala. Whether these various changes are the cause or the result of depression is not entirely certain, but studies in adolescents with depression by Kelly Botteron and other scientists indicate that some changes are likely to be present very early in the disorder. At first glance, this may seem like depressing news for depressed patients—their brains are not the same as those of persons without depression, and depression itself may be bad for their brains.

However, the ability to identify circuitry involved in the disorder offers hope for identifying causes and better treatments. As will be discussed later, there is also hope based on the known effects of some currently available treatments that promote the growth and development of new neurons in part of the hippocampus. Hence effective treatment may help to diminish the effects of the structural changes just described. Finally, based on neuroimaging findings in the PFC, Helen Mayberg and colleagues have taken the bold step of targeting the subgenual anterior cingulate cortex for deep brain stimulation (DBS) in patients with highly refractory (unresponsive to treatment) depressive illness. The results, though still very preliminary, are encouraging and represent a new vista for the field in which neuroimaging has paved the way to a potentially novel form of psychiatric treatment.

Progress is also being made in psychotic disorders such as schizophrenia. Somewhat akin to the findings on major depression, there is evidence for structural changes in several brain regions in people with schizophrenia. These changes include diminished volume of the hippocampus and structural changes in the PFC. Based on work by Francine Benes, David Lewis, and other investigators, there also appears to be a decrease in certain types of inhibitory interneurons in some regions of the schizophrenic brain. Interneurons are generally small neurons that help to regulate local activity in regions of the brain, and they typically communicate with other neurons that are fairly close by. Inhibitory interneurons use the neurotransmitter GABA to decrease the excitability of the principal ("pyramidal") neurons that use glutamate as their neurotransmitter. The relative lack of these inhibitory interneurons in schizophrenia may explain some of the psychotic or cognitive symptoms that patients with this disorder experience, including dysfunction in the PFC and hippocampus.

These findings are already having an impact on the development of new treatment strategies for schizophrenia that target the GABA or glutamate systems. Although these studies are in their infancy, they represent new directions based on the advancing biology of the illness. The traditional target for treating schizophrenia has been the dopamine system. Almost all currently available antipsychotic medications block the function of a specific type of dopamine receptor. Based in part on the effectiveness of these medications, there is a lot of interest in understanding whether there is something wrong with the dopamine system in schizophrenia. This work has produced substantial insight into how dopamine helps to regulate the function of the PFC and working memory and how we filter out unnecessary information when we are trying to concentrate on something. It remains less clear, however, whether a defect in dopamine is a cause or effect of schizophrenia.

Stress and Psychiatric Disorders

It is a popular notion that "stress" causes psychiatric disorders. This is a complicated proposition from many standpoints, not the least of which involves the meanings of the words *stress* and *cause*. In its most generic sense, the statement is a truism; in fact, DSM-IV includes stress-related diagnoses such as acute stress disorder and post-traumatic stress disorder (PTSD). Additionally, there is a lot of scientific interest in the role of stress in producing certain mood disorders, such as major depression. As already emphasized, it is clear that environmental variables are important contributors to the development of psychiatric disorders. Therefore, it seems logical that "stressful" environments are likely to contribute more to these disorders than are "nonstressful" environments. The problem is determining what constitutes a "stressful environment." What is stressful for one person may not be stressful for another (e.g., public speaking); thus, stress appears to reflect both internal and external factors that are unique to each individual. Nonetheless, there is no doubt that certain experiences are stressful for nearly all humans (e.g., death of a loved one).

Much effort has gone into investigating how animals and people respond to both one-time acute stressors and longer-term chronic stressors. Responses to stress include a diverse set of physiological and behavioral changes and are defined by how an organism perceives and reacts to that stress. Stress responses are characterized by a high degree of emotional and physiological arousal under conditions that an individual experiences as negative ("aversive" in scientific terminology). A key component of stress seems to be whether the individual can control the experience. It is a lack of control that often makes a situation stressful.

Through the efforts of a number of scientists, including pioneers such as Hans Selye and modern scientists such as Bruce McEwen, Robert Sapolsky, and others, we have learned a good deal about how the brain and body react to stress. There are clear neurochemical and hormonal changes that help an animal cope initially with stress, but over time these changes result in major adverse effects on the body and brain. Bruce McEwen has championed the term *allostasis* to describe how the body changes its "set point" in response to stress. In other words, the body adjusts its functions and activity in an upward or downward direction depending on the "stress load" it is carrying. Over time, it appears that chronic stress results in wear and tear on the body (termed *allostatic load*), and at times these changes are overwhelming. Under such circumstances, a person suffers increased susceptibility to a variety of medical problems, including altered cardiovascular, metabolic, immune, and neuropsychiatric function. Chronic stress is clearly bad for the brain and results in shrinkage of neurons within the hippocampus, increased susceptibility of regions of the brain to damage and nerve-cell death, and impairments in the generation of new neurons. A culprit in much of this response is the stress hormone cortisol. This hormone promotes acute adaptations to stress but with prolonged exposure and high levels becomes an agent of harm. Behavioral manifestations may include chronic anxiety, heightened and out-of-proportion responses to further stress, and impairments in memory and learning. The role of chronic stress in producing some of the structural changes in the brains of patients with major depression and schizophrenia is an important area for continued investigation. Because of the adverse effects of stress, it seems clear that stress management should play an important role in the treatment of all psychiatric disorders.

Brain Development and Psychiatry

Another area of psychiatric neuroscience that is poised to make major advances involves research into how the development of our brains, both during the prenatal period and in the postnatal years of childhood and adolescence, influences the development and course of psychiatric disorders. Recall our discussion about the role of genes and environment in the cause of these disorders. Many critical genes and critical gene–environment interactions influence how the brain develops to maturity. Thus, a lot of scientific effort is directed toward understanding how genetic changes and events during prenatal and postnatal development influence brain structure and function as we grow. This work is potentially of great relevance to understanding disorders such as schizophrenia and major depression. For example, in early-onset schizophrenia, recent genetic studies have found evidence for novel and rare structural changes in genes that regulate brain development. These structural gene changes involve what are called "copy number variations" (meaning microdeletions or microduplications of segments of specific genes regulating how the brain matures). How these genetic changes occur is not certain but represents an area of intense scientific interest. In studies of individuals at risk for depression, investigators Avshalom Caspi and Terrie Moffitt have identified specific genetic changes (called "polymorphisms") in proteins that transport the neurotransmitter serotonin. These are the same serotonin transporters that are blocked by the antidepressants known as "selective serotonin reuptake inhibitors." But merely inheriting the genetic polymorphism is not enough to result in depression during adulthood; individuals who inherit the genetic predisposition and who also experience stressful life events (e.g., trauma and abuse) are the ones at greatest risk for depression. Other similar examples include polymorphisms affecting the norepinephrine system in individuals at risk for antisocial (criminal and socially deviant) behaviors. Importantly, these studies are starting to identify specific environmental variables that work in concert with specific genetic changes to result in illness. This work is in its infancy, and a recently published analysis of the serotonin transporter findings suggested a need for caution in interpreting the results until further study has been done.

Although many major psychiatric disorders can occur in children, the first manifestations of psychiatric disorder more commonly appear in late adolescence or early adulthood. In some cases, onset may be delayed until much later in adulthood. It is unclear whether (and perhaps unlikely that) the same genetics and gene–environment interactions are involved at the various life stages during which psychiatric disorders can occur. Even for individuals with earlier ages of onset, it is likely that the changes responsible for a disorder are set in motion well before symptoms are detectable. As exemplified by the Caspi and Moffitt studies, current efforts are examining the effects of early childhood abuse and neglect on brain structure and function. Based on the synaptic plasticity story, it appears that even nonabusive adverse events can negatively affect development.

In addition, there are risks associated with certain drug exposures during pre- or postnatal development. For neurons in the brain to survive and develop, they must be appropriately activated (stimulated). But as John Olney and other investigators have shown in their studies of the developing rodent brain, exposure to certain drugs that inhibit neuronal activity leads to dramatic and excessive destruction of developing neurons. This drug-related destruction of developing cells can influence subsequent learning and behavior. A scary part of this story is that the drugs that destroy neurons need only be present for several hours during the time that neurons are first making their synaptic connections with other neurons. In humans, the time that nerve cells would be most susceptible to these effects is during the later part of prenatal gestation and in the first several years of postnatal life. Drugs that have been related to such effects in rodents include certain legal and illegal drugs of abuse, such as alcohol and phencyclidine (PCP), as well as certain clinically used agents, such as anticonvulsants (used to treat epilepsy), sedatives, and anesthetics (used for surgeries). Presently, it is not clear how and whether the effects observed in rodents extend to humans. However, the development of the human brain is a long-term process, particularly when one considers the time it takes for our highest centers in the PFC to mature. Full development of the PFC may not be complete until sometime in early adulthood. Thus, the ability of the drugs just mentioned to damage the developing brain raises great concern about the long-term consequences of repeated and prolonged drug exposure during childhood and adolescence on the development of our highest cognitive processes, such as judgment, planning, and behavioral control. On the other hand, the developing nervous system is incredibly plastic and can adapt to even major insults. In the case of the rodents exposed to the above-mentioned drugs during development, the longer-term defects in their learning and memory are relatively subtle compared to the degree of brain damage experienced. This leads to hope that, for humans, early and targeted interventions, including environmental manipulations, may help to overcome the negative drug effects experienced during development.

Take-Home Messages

- The human brain is complex and reflects the effects of human evolution. Our brains consist of multiple systems that have evolved from and build on the nervous systems of simpler organisms. The highest and most recently evolved levels of our brains give us the capacity for abstract thought and emotional control.

- The human mind is a product of the human brain. Mind reflects brain activity. Like the brain itself, the systems underlying the human mind reflect an assortment of ancient evolutionary systems in combination with newer additions. The primitive systems can override the newer systems, and it takes effort for the newer systems to control the ancient systems. Thus, our emotions are not always under our cognitive control, and cognitive control over emotions can be very hard work.

- Psychiatric disorders are dysfunctions of the mind. Thus, understanding the biology of psychiatric disorders hinges on understanding how the brain allows humans to think, use their emotions, and motivate themselves.

- Our brains function very well as detectors of coincident events, and the plasticity of our synapses (the ability of synapses to change the strength of their connections) reflects this coincidence detection. Coincidence, however, does not mean cause, so our ability to detect and process coincidences does not mean that the inferences drawn by our brains are correct in a causal sense. Furthermore, when our brain gets incomplete information, it tends to fill in the blanks, rightly or wrongly. This type of complexity may have a major role in determining why psychiatric dysfunction is so common. Nonetheless, the remarkable plasticity of our brains is a major plus. In plasticity lies the hope of resilience, effective treatment, and prevention.

- Structural and synaptic changes occur in the brains of people with major psychiatric disorders. Neuroscience is now providing significant insights into these changes. Understanding this biology gives great hope for developing new, more mechanistically based treatments for psychiatric disorders. The advent of deep brain stimulation for highly refractory depression is an early but hopeful outgrowth of this effort.

···*seven*···

How Are Psychiatric Disorders Treated? Basic Principles

Psychiatrists use many different approaches to treat mental disorders. These range from various forms of psychotherapy (talk therapy), patient education, and social interventions to medications and brain stimulation techniques. All of these treatments are important tools, and each can be highly effective and lifesaving in certain situations. In this chapter, we will discuss some basic principles regarding the treatment of psychiatric disorders. In Chapter 8, we will discuss the use of medications. Psychotherapies and lifestyle interventions will be considered in Chapter 9. In Chapter 10, we will review brain stimulation techniques and their use in treating psychiatric disorders. These are all complex topics, and it is beyond the scope of this book to describe specific treatments in detail. Instead, we will present a general overview of the various treatments and their place in psychiatry. For more detailed descriptions of treatment approaches, readers are referred to several excellent sources listed in the bibliography, including the latest editions of *Kaplan and Sadock's Comprehensive Textbook of Psychiatry* and *The American Psychiatric Publishing Textbook of Psychiatry* by Hales, Yudofsky, and Gabbard.

Seven Basic Principles

The basic principles underlying effective psychiatric treatment include the following:

1. *Accurate diagnosis is fundamental to determining appropriate treatment.* The physician's primary goal during the initial interview with any patient is to gather enough information to determine a reasonable working diagnosis of the underlying illness. As discussed earlier, this history gathering may take several interviews and may draw on information not only from the patient but also from others who know the patient well. History gathering is an ongoing process, and doctors often review their thinking concerning the accuracy of their diagnoses. Identifying a diagnosis helps all members of a patient's treatment team know what to expect in terms of the natural progression of the disorder and how the disorder is likely to respond to treatment. Knowing the correct diagnosis also helps the doctor select the best treatments and allows the team to coordinate optimal care. Even when the initial choice of medication is the same for two different diagnoses, it is important to know what to expect over time in terms of the course of the illness. For example, the initial drug treatment for both schizophrenia and mania may involve an antipsychotic medication, but the treatment approaches to each illness over time may be very different.

2. *It is important that the treatment team and the patient stay in close contact.* The care and concern of a treatment team can be very therapeutic. It is normal for patients to feel better knowing that their disorder has a name (i.e., diagnosis) and that concerned health care providers are trying to help them. Even when a patient has a disorder that is very difficult to treat, the fact that professionals are concerned and involved makes a difference. In addition, among the health care professionals who may be involved in a patient's care—for example, psychiatrists, internists, neurologists, psychologists, social workers, nurses, physician's assistants, and counselors—someone needs to be the "point person" who knows in detail what's going on with the patient and who keeps track of the patient's interactions with the various members of the treatment team. This person is usually the psychiatrist, but others can also serve in this role. It is also the point person's responsibility to maintain open lines of communication with the patient, although all members of the team should be

effective communicators. Care can become highly fragmented and frustrating when communications falter within the treatment group and with the patients and their families. Thus, it is critical that patients and their families know who the point person is and feel comfortable about their interactions with that person.

3. *Some symptoms require more aggressive action than others.* Although a patient may suffer from a variety of psychiatric symptoms, some symptoms may elicit more aggressive responses than others. For example, depression is painful, but as long as the risk of self-harm or harm to others is low, then outpatient treatment is usually appropriate. However, some symptoms are medical emergencies and require immediate action to protect the patient and others. A person with schizophrenia who is responding to voices telling him to hurt family members needs emergency care. Hospitalization is necessary in order to protect all concerned. Once the imminent danger has subsided, treatment may continue in a less restrictive environment such as a day hospital or an outpatient setting. Sometimes the patient may not understand why such immediate emergency action is needed; however, friends and family usually support the decision.

4. *Things take time.* Many treatments in psychiatry take a while to work. Although some people with severe symptoms feel better within a few days after starting treatment, most major and sustained responses take weeks to months to occur. This is true whether the treatments are medications, psychotherapies, or other approaches. It is important for patients and families to understand this fact and not to hold unrealistic expectations about the time needed for various treatments to take effect.

5. *The effective use of medications requires expertise on the part of the practitioner.* Medications can be very helpful in treating various psychiatric disorders, especially when used in combination with other types of treatment, including psychotherapies and lifestyle interventions. But effective drug therapy has its own set of principles of which patients and families should be aware, among them:

   a. Every time a medication is prescribed, the physician is making a risk-benefit decision and should involve the patient in this decision. Although medications can have substantial benefits, they can also present definite medical risks depending on many patient-specific factors. Medications should never be prescribed casually.

   b. Most psychiatric medications take several weeks to a few months before their full benefit is observed. Simply put, the brain takes a while to respond to these treatments. This delay can be extremely frustrating for patients and treatment teams alike, and sometimes, the treating physician will prescribe multiple medications or high doses of a medication in an effort to speed things up. Occasionally, short-term treatment with several medications may be appropriate; however, it is becoming increasingly common for patients to be treated initially with three or four medications for the same disorder and then to be kept on all these medications long term. This practice can lead to higher risks from drug interactions and side effects and can be expensive, often with little positive effect; that is, often such polypharmacy neither speeds up recovery nor leads to improved outcome.

c. Patients should inform all their physicians about all the medications that they are taking. Medications can interact with each other and with other illnesses that a patient may have. For example, some psychiatric medications may make diabetes more difficult to control. Also, an internist, if unaware that a patient is taking a certain psychiatric drug, may inadvertently prescribe, for a different illness, a medication that could interact adversely with the psychiatric drug. Moreover, drugs interact in many ways. For instance, one way that medications are eliminated from the body involves the action of the liver. If a new medication is taken that influences how the liver handles those other medications, it can lead to changes in their amount in the body. Sometimes drug levels may increase and cause side effects. Sometimes the new drug may lead to decreased levels of the other drugs and diminish their effectiveness. In addition, different drugs can have direct effects on the same body organs, and the sum of multiple drug effects on some body organs can be unhealthy. These interactions can sometimes directly influence the brain, but they also can influence the heart, liver, blood cells, and other organs.

d. Medications should only be prescribed by a licensed physician or an approved designee of a physician (e.g., a physician's assistant). Currently, there is a movement in some states to allow psychologists or other mental health professionals to prescribe psychiatric medications. We believe strongly that this is a dangerous idea. Psychiatrists learn how to safely prescribe medications as a result of extensive training during four years of medical school and another four years of residency training. In addition, they must meet rigorous state requirements for continuing medical education throughout their careers. Effectively prescribing medications requires knowledge about the various organs of the body, skill in interpreting laboratory tests, and expertise concerning the nature of medical illnesses. Even experienced physicians sometimes have trouble figuring out what is going on when something unexpected happens with a patient during a trial of a medication; those without a formal medical education would have a much harder time dealing with these complexities. This can be dangerous for the patient.

e. Medications should be only one part of a comprehensive treatment approach. Outcomes are better when medications are used in combination with careful follow-up and coordinated care. For those with psychiatric disorders, interpersonal interaction, whether in formal psychotherapy or in informal doctor–patient discussions, is always part of good care.

6. *Types of treatment should be tailored to the patient's individual circumstances.* Depending on the nature of the illness, various types of treatments, as well as their specific sequence, may prove to be useful. For instance, if a patient has schizophrenia and is unable to take care of him- or herself because hallucinations and delusions interfere with basic functioning, the first phase of treatment usually involves protecting the patient in a safe hospital environment while attempting to decrease the severity of the psychotic symptoms with antipsychotic medications. During this early period of treatment, intensive job training would not be appropriate. However, as the patient starts to respond to the first stages of treatment, psychological and social approaches can be helpful. For example, members of the treatment team can start to help the patient learn how to manage basic activities of daily living. As the patient develops better understanding and insight, the treatment team can discuss with him or her the importance of interacting with other people and the importance of avoiding illicit drugs. Once the person is doing better still, various group therapy discussions might prove useful. Also, the patient may benefit from involvement in vocational programs or in a "clubhouse" setting where job skills are taught. Ultimately, each patient has unique circumstances that must be considered when designing the most appropriate overall treatment plan.

7. *As much as possible, patients should be involved in their own care.* Whenever possible, patients and their primary support system (families and friends) should be an important part of the mental health

team. At times, an illness will rob a patient of the ability to understand exactly what is going on around him or her, and it will therefore fall to family and friends to play a critical role in ensuring the patient's care. However, as the patient's symptoms improve and insight returns, he or she can begin to participate in treatment decisions. The more all parties are able to participate effectively in this process, the more likely the treatment will be successful. This collaboration involving the treatment team, the patient, and his or her primary support system builds trust, which is especially important during times of psychiatric crisis. For example, if a patient with bipolar disorder, upon entering a manic phase, loses the ability to recognize that he or she is getting sick, a gut belief in the treatment team may allow the patient to trust their judgment and accept their recommendations for treatment. But involvement in one's own care also carries the responsibility of following through with these recommendations. No treatment plan works when it is not followed; even an absolutely perfect "cure" does not work when it remains in the medication bottle. If patients stop or alter their treatment, they should be honest and let their physicians know. Deciding when and how to change treatment strategies can be complicated, but is predicated on an open and honest dialogue between patients and their doctors.

Evidence-Based Treatments

In the brief overviews that we present in the next few chapters, we focus as much as possible on treatments for which there is the greatest clinical research support. The "gold standard" for making such assessments is the rigorous double-blind, placebo-controlled clinical trial. This means a treatment study in which neither the patient nor the research team knows what type of treatment the patient is getting ("double blind") and in which the active treatment is compared to what is thought to be an inactive treatment (called a "placebo," or "sugar pill" in the popular vernacular). There can be other studies that are "double blind" but not placebo controlled. These studies are usually designed to compare one active treatment to another active treatment in order to determine whether one is more effective than the other. Sometimes, this type of study design is necessary for ethical reasons. For instance, it would be unethical to run placebo-controlled trials with study participants whose condition would become irreversibly worse without active treatment (i.e., for those participants who belonged to the placebo group). But one weakness of the trials that are not placebo controlled is that if they show that both treatments appear equally effective, the researcher can't be certain that either treatment is actually more effective than a placebo. In this case, one would need to assume from earlier work that the active treatment is always more effective than a placebo. In psychiatric trials, this may not be a correct assumption. The current state of science is that many of the treatments in psychiatry have been studied in well-designed clinical trials; others, however, have been less intensively studied or have proven difficult to study. This does not mean that those treatments are ineffective or useless, but only that those treatments have less data to support them. There are "treatments" in psychiatry, however, that are ineffective and probably harmful; we try to point those out along the way in subsequent chapters.

We also want to make a few comments about placebo effects in psychiatry. Some mental disorders include a lot of psychological symptoms (e.g., sadness, guilt) that often improve as soon as the patients receive attention. Thus, in clinical trials of treatments for psychiatric disorders such as depression, there can be a high degree of "placebo response." That is, simply being enrolled in the study, interacting with concerned individuals, and having an expectation of improvement can produce benefits for many patients in these trials. We estimate that about a third of the patients enrolled in studies of depression treatment exhibit placebo responses. Typically, these types of responses are shorter lived than the responses that occur with active treatment, but distinguishing active from placebo responses can be very difficult. Additionally, just because patients may have a placebo response doesn't mean they have had an artificial response. In very well done studies of treatments for a variety of neurological, medical, and psychiatric disorders, significant placebo responses occurred that often involved specific changes in the brain. For example, there is a high placebo response in certain pain states, and some studies have shown that these responses involve actual changes in the brain systems underlying pain perception. Similarly, Parkinson's disease, a neurodegenerative illness, also has a significant placebo response rate, and those responses involve changes in the brain's dopamine system, the same system that is undergoing degeneration from the disease. To us, these placebo responses point out how resilient the human brain is and how human expectations can sometimes foster self-healing. Harnessing these capabilities might eventually help in the design of better treatments in the future.

Take-Home Messages

- There are many options available for treating psychiatric disorders. All can produce significant benefits but can also be associated with side effects. The choice of treatment should always result from a collaborative discussion between the doctor and the patient and should take into account a careful analysis of the risk-benefit ratio.

- By becoming educated consumers, patients and their families can greatly facilitate all medical care. Understanding symptoms of disorders, the options for treatments, and the time course that is required for clinical benefits is part of what it means to be an educated consumer. Being open and honest with treatment team members is part of what it means to be a responsible one.

··· eight ···

Medications

A comprehensive discussion of psychotropic medications, now the mainstays in the management of most psychiatric disorders, is beyond the scope of this book. We believe, however, that a brief survey of various categories of psychiatric medications may be helpful for patients and families. The general principles outlined in the previous chapter pertain to each of these groups of medications.

Antidepressants

Since the advent of Prozac (fluoxetine) and its popularization in the media, antidepressants have become the class of psychotropic medications most familiar to the general public. The most common group of antidepressants is known as the SSRIs (*selective serotonin reuptake inhibitors*). Examples of SSRIs include household names like Prozac (fluoxetine), Paxil (paroxetine), Zoloft (sertraline), Celexa (citalopram), Lexapro (escitalopram), and Luvox (fluvoxamine). Increasingly, these medications are available in generic forms, resulting in lower costs to patients than in the past. The name *SSRI* comes from the action that these medications exert on a brain chemical called serotonin. Serotonin is a neurotransmitter that is released from the end of certain nerve cells and influences nearby nerve cells. It is subsequently removed from the space between the cells by a type of molecular "pump" called the "serotonin transporter." SSRIs interfere with the function of the serotonin transporter, thus increasing the amount of serotonin left in the space between cells. Interestingly, although this effect on the transporter occurs very quickly, SSRIs take several weeks to work. Why? It is likely that the antidepressant effect of SSRIs requires long-term changes in nerve cells that are initiated by the transporter blockade and the resulting increases in serotonin levels in specific regions of the brain. These long-term changes eventually influence the activity of genes in certain neurons. These genes may influence the survival, growth, and patterns of connections of certain nerve cells.

During the first week or two after the initiation of SSRI treatment, people may notice little improvement in their symptoms, but they may experience side effects such as mild stomach upset or increased nervousness. These early side effects usually go away, and in time, the medications usually do help people feel better from both depressive symptoms and symptoms of anxiety. For reasons that aren't fully understood, young people may experience an increase in impulsive thoughts, including thoughts of suicide, early in treatment with these medications. This reaction seems to occur most often in adolescent patients and is less common when people reach their twenties. Often, it is difficult to determine whether the impulsivity is a result of the medications or the underlying psychiatric disorder. Regardless, careful monitoring of younger patients by the treatment team is especially important during the early phases of treatment.

The dose of medication that a patient is prescribed initially may not be the dose that is eventually effective. The treatment team often works with the patient to increase the dose gradually over the first month or so. One reason that lower doses of medications are used early in treatment is to diminish the risk of side effects and to determine the lowest dose that works for a given patient. With these medications, as with all psychiatric medications, more is often not better, and starting with too high of an initial dose or raising doses too quickly can lead to unnecessary complications, bad outcomes, and patient dissatisfaction.

At the time that SSRIs (and other antidepressants) are started, the treatment team has to decide whether to use the medications alone or to initiate more formal psychotherapy as well. These decisions are made in collaboration with the patient. Some patients prefer to see if the medications (along with close monitoring) work well enough alone, without combining it initially with psychotherapy. For patients to do well with this drug treatment approach, they must continue to take the medications for an extended period of time. If they feel well after eight weeks or so of treatment and then stop the medication, thinking that the illness is "cured," they are very likely to relapse quickly.

To avoid this problem, the treatment team typically counsels patients about the overall expected length of treatment. This varies depending on each individual's previous history. If this is a patient's first episode of depression and the family history doesn't include significant depression, the patient may be able to slowly decrease and then stop the medications after about 6 to 12 months of doing well. The word *slowly* is very important. Should symptoms start to return, then the dose can be returned to the therapeutic level. Should a person stop medications, do well for several years, and then have another episode, chances are good that he or she will respond to medication treatment again. In such instances, continuing the medications for a longer period than before may be considered. Some people have only one or two episodes of depression during their lives; however, it is common that people have a larger number of lifetime episodes. Some people have chronic symptoms of depression, although such symptoms may vary in intensity over time. Longer-term (meaning years) and even life-long use of antidepressant medications can be helpful in such cases to maintain benefits and avoid relapses. Similarly, individuals with frequent recurrences of depression may require life-long treatment.

A significant minority of patients on SSRIs experience sexual dysfunction, including decreased ability to achieve orgasm. It is possible that as the depression improves sexual drive and performance may also improve and even be enhanced. Psychiatrists will typically ask about sexual side effects of SSRIs, and patients should feel free to discuss this issue with the treatment team. The risks and benefits of trying a different medication can be explored, and just because a patient experiences a particular side effect with one medication doesn't mean that he or she will necessarily have the same side effect with a different medication.

As mentioned, other side effects of SSRIs can include upset stomach and jitteriness, particularly early in treatment. These can often be managed with reassurance or low doses of an appropriate antinausea or antianxiety medication. It should, however, be mentioned that some SSRIs, particularly Prozac, can have powerful interactions with other medicines. Such interactions can influence the effectiveness and safe use of other medications. For this reason, patients should tell their doctors about *all* the medications they are taking, including over-the-counter drugs such as antihistamines, cold remedies, and sleeping pills.

SSRIs are not addictive drugs, but some patients may experience odd effects if they stop these medications (and other antidepressants) suddenly. Such effects can include peculiar sensations, headaches, and "popping" (electrical-like sensations) in their heads. These symptoms usually go away if the patient restarts the medication and are less bothersome when the medication is discontinued slowly over weeks or months.

Another group of antidepressant medications is known as SNRIs (*sero-tonin and norepinephrine reuptake inhibitors*). Effexor (venlafaxine), Cymbalta (duloxetine), and Pristiq (desvenlafaxine) are in this category. These medications may block the reuptake transporters of two neurotransmitters, serotonin and norepinephrine. Once again, the effect of blocking these transporters is very quick, yet the drugs take weeks to work. The long-term influence of these drugs on the genetic machinery of cells may be very similar to the effects of the SSRIs. SNRIs may have somewhat different side effects than SSRIs, but the same points discussed before hold for all the antidepressants.

Patients sometimes wonder why different classes of antidepressants (and other medications) are needed and how their physicians select among the various classes. It is important to have a variety of medications from which to choose because patients differ in their reaction to specific medications in terms of treatment response and side effects. Even though the effectiveness of any one group of antidepressants is about equal to any other group, individual patients are likely to have a particular medication that works best for them. Sometimes the choice of initial medication is based on the likely side effects that will be encountered and on the physician's assessment of how well the patient will tolerate them.

One drug that seems to work differently than either the SSRIs or the SNRIs is Wellbutrin (bupropion). We don't really understand how this drug works; some studies suggest that it influences the dopamine neurotransmitter that is involved in many brain functions, including the central reward system, but this is far from certain. In addition to its actions as an antidepressant, bupropion can be beneficial for smokers who are attempting to quit smoking. The nicotine in cigarettes stimulates the central reward system, and bupropion helps regulate this system during nicotine withdrawal.

Interestingly, sexual side effects do not seem to be as much of a problem with bupropion. Also, the weight gain some people experience with certain antidepressants isn't usually seen with bupropion. It does have its own spectrum of side effects, however. For instance, bupropion, especially at higher doses, increases the risk for seizures. This side effect is of particular concern for people predisposed to seizures, as well as for people suffering from certain eating disorders. The reason patients with eating disorders are at increased risk for seizures is not certain, but it may reflect changes in metabolism associated with the primary psychiatric disorder. Bupropion, like other medications, requires dose adjustment, which must be done carefully to avoid the risks of seizures. Thus, treatment with bupropion should be monitored carefully by a physician.

Remeron (mirtazapine) is a relatively new antidepressant medication. It has a somewhat unique mechanism of action, inhibiting certain serotonin and norepinephrine receptors. Receptors are proteins on the surface of nerve cells that allow specific neurotransmitters to exert their influence on the cells. Because of effects on a certain serotonin receptor, mirtazapine helps to decrease nausea and gastric distress; this can be a helpful "side effect" for patients who suffer from both depression and gastrointestinal or other medical illnesses. Remeron can be sedating, however, and weight gain can be another significant side effect.

Desyrel (trazodone) and Serzone (nefazodone) are other antidepressant medications that inhibit certain serotonin receptors. They also have weak effects on serotonin transporters. Desyrel can be very sedating, and in doses lower than needed to treat depression, it is sometimes used to promote sleep. It has been associated with certain rare but severe side effects, including prolonged penile erections in men that may require medical intervention to reverse. Serzone has been associated with rare but potentially serious liver and cardiac problems. Thus, neither agent is commonly used as an antidepressant anymore.

We also want to mention two other groups of antidepressants that are important for historical reasons and are still in clinical use today. Tricyclic antidepressants (TCAs) and monoamine oxidase inhibitors (MAOIs) are the oldest antidepressants; MAOIs were the first category of antidepressants available for clinical use. They both act by increasing the availability of norepinephrine and serotonin, but they do so by different mechanisms: TCAs inhibit the reuptake transporters for these neurotransmitters, while MAOIs increase the availability of these neurotransmitters by blocking their chemical destruction by the body. Examples of TCAs include Elavil (amitriptyline), Tofranil (imipramine), Pamelor (nortriptyline), and Norpramin (desipramine). Currently available MAOIs include Nardil (phenelzine), Parnate (tranylcypromine), and Marplan (isocarboxazid). Deprenyl (selegiline) is another MAOI used to treat Parkinson's disease. This medication was not thought initially to have antidepressant effects, but this was found to be dose-related, and so a form of selegiline (Ensam) is now available as a skin patch for treating depression.

Both TCAs and MAOIs can be effective but have much more prominent side effects than the antidepressants described previously. Thus, their use is best supervised by a knowledgeable psychiatrist. Indeed, MAOIs aren't used very often because patients must avoid certain foods and medications when taking them. There are, however, some patients who don't respond to other antidepressants but who have a very good response to the MAOIs. Why do the MAOIs require substantial dietary restrictions? In addition to blocking the destruction of neurotransmitters in the brain, MAOIs also block the destruction of certain chemicals in the gut. One of these chemicals, tyramine, is found in many foods, including several common cheeses. If tyramine isn't destroyed in the gut, it can enter the bloodstream and cause a sudden, large release of transmitters such as norepinephrine. This can lead to a sudden, dramatic, and dangerous surge in blood pressure called a "hypertensive crisis." There are many foods that must be avoided by people taking MAOIs, and psychiatrists who prescribe these drugs will review the list of foods with their patients.

Similarly, many medications, including some sold over the counter, can interact with MAOIs and lead to a similar surge in blood pressure. Another syndrome, called the "serotonin syndrome," can occur when MAOIs interact with other drugs that increase serotonin, such as the SSRIs. This syndrome can influence blood pressure regulation and has neurologic consequences (e.g., tremors and twitching movements called "myoclonus"). It is understandable that many doctors are not big fans of MAOIs. Nevertheless, some patients respond so well to them that it is important for psychiatrists to have this type of drug available as a treatment option.

Mood Stabilizers

Mood stabilizers are the first line of treatments for people suffering with bipolar disorder. These medications can be helpful for manic symptoms, depressive symptoms, or a mixture of both. The three types of mood stabilizers most often used are lithium, mood-stabilizing anticonvulsants, and antipsychotic medications. Antidepressant medications, although sometimes used to treat the depressive phase of bipolar disorder, may not be as effective as once thought. Recent data suggest that there are few long-lasting benefits from antidepressant medications in bipolar patients and that sometimes antidepressants may contribute to instability in the longer-term clinical course of the illness, including increased periods of mania. Data on this topic are still limited, however, and patients should work closely with their doctors to decide the appropriate course of treatment.

Lithium is a chemical that can alleviate both the manic and depressive phases of bipolar disorder. It has been available for decades and can be lifesaving in terms of decreasing symptoms and suicide risk. Many nonpsychiatric physicians prefer that psychiatrists undertake the prescribing and management of lithium, perhaps because the drug can have significant side effects, especially when the dose is too high. Fortunately, there is a close relationship between the beneficial effects and blood levels of lithium. For this reason, lithium levels in the blood are typically measured several times during the beginning months of treatment. Once a therapeutic level is achieved and symptoms are stable, drug levels may be measured about twice a year. Lithium can sometimes influence kidney and thyroid function, and so physicians periodically order simple blood tests to monitor these functions.

Many patients find lithium very easy to tolerate; others are bothered by a feeling of being slowed down or blunted. Some report the need to urinate more often, and some notice a slight hand tremor. Interestingly, even though many patients with bipolar disorder recognize that mood stabilizers such as lithium help them tremendously, they feel that these drugs tend to rob them of the exciting feeling that comes from a manic episode. Mania can feel good at first, and it can be a real challenge to convince patients who are feeling good during a manic episode that they should take medications that will make them feel less "high." Even patients who are doing well on lithium will sometimes decide to stop taking their medicines for several days. They start to feel good off the medications and rapidly lose insight about why they need treatment. The disorder can then quickly cycle out of control, and before long, the good feeling of mania can rapidly deteriorate to irritability and erratic behavior.

Lithium can interact with certain medications, and so doctors need to know about all medications that their patients are taking, including over-the-counter drugs. There are also special considerations for women who are taking lithium during pregnancy. A similar statement can be made about most mood stabilizers, and, therefore, women with bipolar disorder who are thinking about becoming pregnant should discuss these issues openly with their doctors.

Exactly how lithium works to relieve the symptoms of bipolar disorder remains a mystery. Lithium is a simple element, but it has many effects on a host of cellular functions in the brain. Among other effects, lithium helps protect nerve cells from destruction and may increase connections between neurons. Examining whether the neuroprotective effects of lithium are related to its benefits in bipolar disorder is an active area of research.

Lithium is a medication that a person may need to take for years or decades. Episodes of bipolar disorder frequently return, and continued use of the medications is necessary to minimize the frequency and severity of these return bouts. As a person hits senior-citizen age, kidney function slows down, and this, in turn, can influence lithium levels in the body. Thus, the dose may need to be adjusted as people enter their 60s or if they develop illnesses that change their kidney function. People should probably think about treatment with lithium the way they think about treatment with drugs used to lower high blood pressure or high cholesterol; that is, once the drug is initiated, it is likely to be continued for the rest of the patients' lives.

Anticonvulsants are a group of drugs used to decrease the frequency of seizures in persons with epilepsy. Several (but not all) anticonvulsants are also excellent mood stabilizers. Three anticonvulsants used to treat bipolar disorder are Depakote (valproic acid), Tegretol (carbamazepine), and Lamictal (lamotrigine). Each of these drugs has its own advantages and disadvantages. They can interact powerfully with other drugs. Measuring blood levels can be useful in regulating the dose of Depakote and Tegretol, although clinical response is the gold standard for determining effectiveness. Because of the potential for severe side effects, a doctor's expertise is necessary to help a patient appropriately manage these medications. Lamictal can cause a type of rash that may indicate a syndrome that can be fatal. Therefore, this drug is usually started at a low dose and slowly increased. If a rash develops, the drug is usually stopped. Interestingly, there is some evidence that Lamictal may have particular benefit in the depressed phase of bipolar disorder. Other anticonvulsants, including Neurontin (gabapentin) and Topamax (topiramate), have been used to treat bipolar disorder, but there are only limited data to support their use for treating this disorder, and their effectiveness, if any, does not appear to match the effectiveness of Depakote, Tegretol, or Lamictal.

Antipsychotic medications, to be discussed in more detail in the next section, can also be helpful as mood stabilizers, especially during the early phase of treatment when psychotic symptoms and agitation can be prominent. There are patients who seem to respond well to antipsychotics long term and who relapse when such a drug is stopped. These drugs can have long-term consequences and, like all drugs, require a careful risk-benefit assessment by patients, their family and friends, and the mental health team.

Frequently, it takes a while to find the best medicine or combination of medications to help people with bipolar disorder. It is easy for doctors and patients to become impatient with this effort and to resort to the simultaneous use of a large number of medications. Sometimes, such polypharmacy is rational, as in prescribing medications with different mechanisms of actions (e.g., combining lithium with an antipsychotic medication) for the initial treatment of a person with agitated or psychotic mania. Sometimes, however, this polypharmacy is irrational; that is, too many drugs are added in a short sequence, making it difficult to know how many are actually needed. Assessments between patients and their doctors about all of the patient's medications should be repeated throughout the course of treatment.

Bipolar disorder has become an increasingly common diagnosis in children and adolescents, and many youngsters with this diagnosis are taking a large number of mood stabilizers. It is understandable that everyone wants to help kids when they are sick. However, little is actually known about the effects of these drugs on the developing brain; at present, the data are limited as to the effectiveness, risks, and benefits of drugs in treating bipolar-like symptoms in young children. It requires a great deal of expertise (usually involving a child psychiatrist) to make this diagnosis accurately and to treat its symptoms effectively. Families should communicate frequently with their doctors to ensure that these medications, especially in combination with other drugs, are used cautiously.

Antipsychotics

This very powerful group of medications is used to treat psychotic symptoms (hallucinations, delusions, and thought disorder) occurring in a variety of illnesses, including schizophrenia, bipolar disorder, psychotic depression, and delirium. These medications can have significant benefits but also can have significant side effects.

The first generation of antipsychotic medications became available in the 1950s. Over time, many first-generation antipsychotics were developed and approved for use. Common names include Thorazine (chlorpromazine), Prolixin (fluphenazine), Mellaril (thioridazine), Navane (thiothixene), and Haldol (haloperidol). They seem to work by blocking the actions of the neurotransmitter dopamine at a specific type of dopamine receptor. These medications revolutionized psychiatric care at the time of their development and contributed to the release of a large number of patients from chronic care facilities known as asylums. Other reasons, some of them political, also contributed to this "deinstitutionalization" movement and led to the eventual closing of many large chronic care facilities. Unfortunately, some patients still require long-term care, but the number of facilities providing this care is now sparse.

The first-generation antipsychotic drugs are associated with numerous side effects, including certain types of movement disorders. One such movement disorder includes features similar to those in Parkinson's disease: rigid muscle tone, slowed movements, and a certain type of resting tremor (called a "pill-rolling tremor" when observed in the hands). Another is called akathesia, which is an uncomfortable internal feeling of restlessness that causes a person to want to pace and move around. Another side effect that some patients develop is a sudden muscle spasm in the neck, causing the patients to hold their heads in an uncomfortable and, at times, dangerous posture. This response is called an "acute dystonic reaction," and it responds rapidly to treatment with drugs like Cogentin (benztropine). Some people taking antipsychotic medications for extended periods of time develop an involuntary chewing motion called "tardive dyskinesia." Movement disorders that develop after years of antipsychotic treatment may or may not reverse when the medication is stopped, and they are among the greatest drawbacks of the early antipsychotic medications. Other side effects of some of these medications include significant weight gain and marked tiredness. Some people also notice that they get dizzy upon standing. This is called "orthostatic hypotension," and it is caused by a lowering of blood pressure for a brief period of time when one stands up.

Thus, although the older medications worked well to diminish active psychotic symptoms in many patients, their significant side effects and risks were problematic. Newer medications were developed in an attempt to improve effectiveness while decreasing the risks. Examples of such medications include Zyprexa (olanzapine), Risperdal (risperidone), Geodon (ziprasidone), Abilify (aripiprazole), and Seroquel (quetiapine). And indeed, these newer ("second-generation") medications were initially thought to be significantly better and safer than the older medicines. They do not, for example, have nearly the degree of movement disorder side effects, so this is a major advantage. As a result, their use rapidly and substantially increased, including for conditions on which the data were inconclusive about their effectiveness. The notion that they have few major side effects, however, has proven to be incorrect.

As we accumulate more data and clinical experience, it is becoming apparent that the newer antipsychotic drugs may not be much more effective than the older drugs, and some can have serious side effects of their own, such as significant weight gain and a deleterious influence on blood sugars and blood fats, possibly leading to diabetes and increased cholesterol and triglyceride levels in the blood. Some of them also, at higher doses, can even cause movement disorders. Yet the fact that younger psychiatrists don't see many of the movement side effects that were common just a few decades ago is an indication of the advantage of the newer drugs. On the other hand, because of the greatly increased use of the newer drugs, we are seeing many more patients with substantial weight gain. In fact, routine monitoring of weight, waist size, and blood sugar is now recommended for patients taking these antipsychotic medications.

The second-generation antipsychotic drugs are also being used in children and younger adolescents. Obesity in all age groups, including and perhaps especially in our youth, is a major problem in our society, and it is important that mental health providers try to avoid adding to this problem. Very careful evaluation of the potential benefits and risks of using these medications in younger patients needs to be made by the treatment team and thoroughly discussed with the family and patient. Data about the metabolic effects of antipsychotic medications in children are lacking.

One antipsychotic medication that may be unique is Clozaril (clozapine). This agent was initially developed in the heyday of the first-generation medications, but it was kept off the market because of major adverse effects on white blood cells (which help to fight infections in the body). Nonetheless, repeated studies demonstrated that Clozaril can help patients with psychotic disorders who do not respond to other antipsychotic drugs and may decrease the risk of suicide in schizophrenia. Thus, in the late 1980s, Clozaril was released for clinical use with specific guidelines about its use and monitoring. Among the antipsychotics, it is the one agent that truly may be "atypical" (a term that has been loosely applied to second-generation antipsychotics in general). It seems to help patients whom no other medications help, and it has a low incidence of causing movement disorders. It does have a number of significant side effects, however, including the potential for effects on white blood counts and the propensity to cause significant weight gain.

Longer-acting versions of some antipsychotic medications are available. Examples include the decanoate forms of haloperidol (Haldol-D) and flu-phenazine (Prolixin-D) and, more recently, a long-acting, injectable form of risperidone (Risperdal), known as Risperdal Consta. These agents are administered by deep-muscle injections, and the active drug is released slowly from the reservoir in muscle. Importantly, these long-acting antipsychotic medications are administered on less frequent schedules (e.g., usually biweekly or monthly instead of daily) and are used to help manage patients whose insight into their illnesses is so impaired that they are noncompliant with routine treatment. The use of these long-acting drugs requires close communication between the treatment team and patients and their families to maintain compliance and to detect side effects when they occur.

The bottom line with antipsychotic medications is that they are powerful drugs that can be lifesaving when used correctly. Sometimes they are needed for short periods of time; often, however, they are used for chronic disorders such as schizophrenia, which may require life-long treatment. In addition, physicians must keep up to date on the different side effects of these drugs in order to work with the patient and the family in choosing the best medication. The older and newer antipsychotics have different side effect profiles. Some of the more recently developed drugs such as Geodon (ziprasidone) or Abilify (aripiprazole) may have better profiles in terms of balancing benefit and risk related to movement disorders and weight gain. Unfortunately, these and the other newer antipsychotics do not have generic versions and are expensive. Whatever medication is ultimately recommended, the treatment team must communicate with the patient and caregivers to ensure that they understand the reasons for the recommended treatment and its likely course. If, however, a mental health provider is recommending antipsychotic medications for mild depression or mild anxiety, it may be prudent for the patient to obtain a second opinion.

Antianxiety Medications

Many antidepressant medications also are effective in treating anxiety, and the SSRIs in particular have become mainstays in the treatment of panic disorder and obsessive-compulsive disorder (OCD). Benzodiazepines are a specific type of antianxiety medications (also known as "anxiolytics") that were introduced into the market beginning in the 1960s. Valium (diazepam), Librium (chlordiazepoxide), Ativan (lorazepam), and Xanax (alprazolam) are four commonly used medications that are classified as benzodiazepines. This group of medications works by increasing the effectiveness of gamma-aminobutyric acid (GABA), a neurotransmitter that usually inhibits or slows down brain cell firing. Benzodiazepines enhance this effect of GABA, causing sedation and relaxation.

Unlike antidepressant drugs, which must be taken for weeks before they work, benzodiazepines can be effective quickly after even a single dose. Thus, they can be useful short term for situational anxiety (e.g., a fear of flying). They can also be useful in the long-term treatment of chronic anxiety disorders (e.g., panic disorder, OCD, general anxiety disorder, and social phobias). They do have their disadvantages, however. Because of their sedative effects, they can interfere with function. At higher doses, they can also dull the senses and a person's ability to think. If a person's senses are on hyperdrive due to anxiety, a slight dulling may not be problematic, but for others, a slight blunting of memory and thinking may be so worrisome as to cancel out any relief from the anxiety. In older persons especially, the sedative effects of these medications can be associated with memory problems and falls—a bad combination that can have markedly adverse effects on function and independence.

Another issue with the benzodiazepines is that higher doses over long periods of time can cause the body to become dependent on them. Here, the term *dependent* means that a person must continue taking the drug in order to avoid an uncomfortable and sometimes dangerous withdrawal reaction. This dependency is less common and less severe than the dependency that occurred in earlier days when barbiturates were used to treat anxiety. In fact, most people taking benzodiazepines for anxiety respond well to the drugs and do not need larger doses as time goes on. Nevertheless, it is important for the prescribing doctor to consider a patient's age, physical health, psychiatric condition, and use of other medications when choosing the best benzodiazepine for a particular person. When the patient and the health care team decide that it is time to decrease or discontinue these medications, it is best to taper the dose slowly. If one were to stop taking high doses of these drugs suddenly, there is a possibility of drug withdrawal reactions that can vary from uncomfortable to dangerous. It also perhaps goes without saying that if a person has a tendency to abuse substances, it is best to stay away from this category of drug altogether.

The various benzodiazepines that are available on the market differ in terms of how long an individual dose stays in the body. They also differ in terms of how the body metabolizes and disposes of them. Withdrawal reactions tend to be more severe for benzodiazepines that stay in the body for shorter periods of time than those that remain for longer periods. Among the shorter-duration drugs are Xanax (alprazolam) and Ativan (lorazepam), while longer-duration drugs include Valium (diazepam) and Klonopin (clonazepam). For example, some patients notice withdrawal effects from Xanax within 8 to 12 hours after their last dose. Symptoms include increased nervousness and tremor, symptoms that feel like worsening anxiety. This can lead to a vicious cycle in which more Xanax is taken at more frequent intervals to combat withdrawal. If patients have such an experience, they should discuss it thoroughly with their doctor because this cycle can lead to marked dependency on the drug.

A very different type of antianxiety agent is called Buspar (buspirone). This drug is neither an antidepressant nor a benzodiazepine and has unique properties, seeming to work by influencing certain subtypes of serotonin receptors. Similar to antidepressants, it does not work quickly and requires weeks of treatment before it becomes effective. It has fewer side effects than many of the antidepressants. It is not habit forming and does not have the same side effects as the benzodiazepines. Still, some doctors think that this medicine is not quite as effective as either of the two other categories of antianxiety drugs. Its antianxiety effect may also be more subtle. Patients who have been treated with benzodiazepines can often tell the difference between their antianxiety effects and those of Buspar.

Medications for Alzheimer's Type Dementia

One of the great stories in clinical neuroscience is the tremendous progress being made in understanding the causes of Alzheimer's disease. It is a devastating illness that robs its victims of their identity; it gradually destroys their memory abilities, thinking abilities, and social abilities—indeed, the illness can change the very elements that constitute personality. Scientists now have a good idea about the processes going wrong in the brain that may lead to these clinical symptoms. Unfortunately, scientific progress has not yet led to the development of powerfully effective therapies, but there is reason to hope that these will become available in the near future. Indeed, if research continues to progress at its current rate, we may be within a decade of having treatments that could substantially slow, if not halt, the disease.

In the meantime, there are two major categories of medications that can delay the progression of the disease at least for a short time. The first category is the cholinesterase inhibitors. These medications increase the effectiveness of a neurotransmitter called acetylcholine, which helps with learning and memory. Aricept (donepezil), Razadyne (galantamine), and Exelon (rivastigmine) are examples of this kind of drug. These medicines do not reverse the brain changes that occur in Alzheimer's disease. They do, however, slow down further changes for about 6 to 12 months. After this time, the disease progresses at about the same rate as before the drug was taken. This delay in disease progression has been shown in people with mild to moderate illness. Some clinicians believe that cholinesterase inhibitors may be able to slow the progression even at the very mild stage of illness.

It is important for doctors to differentiate normal age-related changes in memory and learning from abnormal changes that represent the beginning of the disease. This is a complex clinical problem, and some medical centers, particularly those that house Alzheimer's Disease Research Centers (ADRCs), are very adept at this distinction. Cholinesterase inhibitors are unlikely to slow normal age-related changes in cognitive function. Even so, we are starting to see these medications prescribed to patients who are referred to as the "worried well." These are older people who are worried about, and perhaps very sensitive to, subtle changes that nonetheless don't suggest the beginnings of Alzheimer's disease. Individuals concerned about age-related changes in cognition are advised to consult centers that specialize in Alzheimer's disease.

The ability of cholinesterase inhibitors to slow progression for 6 to 12 months, although helpful, is only a small step in dealing with Alzheimer's disease. The medications are costly and can have significant side effects, including gastrointestinal distress. One can ask whether even such a small effect is worth the cost. This is a question that doctors, patients, and families need to ask and answer together. A person with mild but definite symptoms who can maintain function for an extra year and who may want that time to watch grandkids develop or to put personal affairs in order may feel that the benefit these medications offer is very important. But a person who has moderate illness—that is, who has reached the stage in the disease where he or she now likely depends on help from others for many basic activities—may not wish to start a medication that might prolong this uncomfortable state of health. This question is just one of a large number of ethical issues that surround the treatment of moderate to advanced Alzheimer's disease.

The other drug that has been shown to help patients with Alzheimer's disease is called Namenda (memantine). It is not known exactly how this drug works, but it appears to influence the glutamate neurotransmitter system via the N-methyl-D-aspartate (NMDA) receptor. These receptors are thought to play a major role in learning and memory, but when excessively activated, they can be associated with a loss of neurons, via a process called "excitotoxicity" (i.e., toxicity resulting from excessive nerve-cell excitation). Namenda has been shown to slow Alzheimer's disease that has reached the moderate stages. It may not be helpful during the very mild or mild stages. While it doesn't reverse symptoms, it, too, may slow disease progression for 6 to 12 months. It seems to work by a different mechanism than the cholinesterase inhibitors, and its effects can be additive with a cholinesterase inhibitor once the moderate stage of illness has been reached. Thus, Namenda can be appropriate for a person taking a cholinesterase inhibitor who has progressed to the moderate stage of illness. Again, the decision to consider slowing progression of this illness once it has reached a moderate stage needs to be made carefully. Ideally, the doctor and family members should discuss these issues with the patient prior to the onset of the moderate stage—that is, at a time when the patient is still able to communicate his or her wishes in such circumstances.

Sleep Medications

Many of us are not satisfied with our sleep, and there are many reasons why we don't sleep well. These include psychiatric illnesses such as depression, alcohol abuse, and anxiety disorders; medical disorders such as sleep apnea (the temporary shutdown of breathing during sleep); stress; and poor sleep hygiene. This last reason for insomnia may be best addressed by using some common sense. For example, sleep experts indicate that our beds and bedrooms should be associated *only* with sleep and intimacy and should not be used for activities such as working on a laptop, playing cards, eating, watching TV, or gabbing away on the phone. Other lifestyle changes can also be very beneficial and are critical first steps in dealing with insomnia. Avoid drinking caffeinated beverages, for example, anytime in the evening. Caffeine is a stimulant; hence ingesting it prior to trying to sleep makes no sense. Nicotine is also a stimulant, and so eliminating cigarette use can have positive effects on sleep (not to mention the benefits that could come from improved breathing during sleep). Some medicines with a stimulant side effect should generally not be taken at bedtime. Alcohol is another agent that can cause sleep problems. Although alcohol is sedating, this effect wears off in a few hours, sometimes leading to wakefulness in the middle of the night or early morning. This early awakening is actually a mild form of acute withdrawal.

Avoiding these substances and improving sleep hygiene can go a long way toward resolving problems with sleep, but they do take personal effort and some discipline. Perhaps for that reason, many people don't implement these techniques, preferring instead to employ quicker fixes from sleep medications. Many drugs are advertised as over-the-counter sleep remedies. Often these drugs are antihistamines that have sedation as a side effect, and some are the same agents used in a number of over-the-counter treatments for common colds, for example, Benadryl (diphenhydramine), an antihistamine. Although the sedating effect may initially help someone fall asleep, in general these medications can have significant side effects, including cognitive impairment. Most doctors would not recommend these medications as a longer-term solution for sleep problems. The sedative effects may decrease over time, and the side effects may be substantial. Persons taking over-the-counter sleep medications on a routine basis should let their doctor know. These drugs can be powerful and can interact with other medicines. It should not be assumed, in other words, that a medication is safe just because it doesn't require a prescription.

Prescription medications that a doctor may recommend for patients diagnosed with serious sleep problems include those that act on GABA receptors to enhance the effects of the neurotransmitter GABA. There are several subtypes of GABA receptors, and benzodiazepines such as Valium (diazepam) enhance many, but not all, of these receptor subtypes. This enhancement is responsible for the various effects of Valium-like drugs, including sedation (sleepiness), antianxiety effects, antiseizure effects, and muscle-relaxant effects (at high doses). Many of these GABA-benzodiazepine receptors are also enhanced by more recently approved sleep medications, such as Lunesta (eszopiclone). Although the chemistry of Lunesta is different from that of the benzodiazepines, it works in very similar ways to them. Ambien (zolpidem) is an example of a drug that targets the specific subtype of GABA receptors responsible for sedation. Thus, this drug is an effective medication for aiding sleep but lacks the antianxiety properties of other benzodiazepine-like drugs.

The benzodiazepine-type sleep medications work quickly and do not need to be taken for a long time before their effect is achieved. They can help a person fall asleep, and depending on the specific drug, some can be effective throughout the night. Some of the benzodiazepines are long acting, meaning that their sedating and antianxiety properties can last a day or more in the body. The sedating properties can as a result lead to hangover-type effects the next day. These medications can have other side effects as well, particularly in the elderly. Excessive sedation, confusion, and falls are some of the possible adverse effects. Moreover, the effects of these medications can be additive with other sedating drugs, including alcohol. These sleep medications should not be taken during the day or at any time when a person is engaged in activities that requires him or her to be fully alert.

Some doctors take advantage of the sedating properties of other medications to help a patient sleep, prescribing, for example, low doses of the antidepressant Desyrel (trazodone) for this purpose. Data demonstrating that this drug is a good sleep aid over long periods of time are lacking, so it is not clear whether its routine use for sleep is justified, although this seems to be an increasingly common practice.

The use of prescription sleep medicines can be very helpful, especially for short-term difficulties with sleep. Unfortunately, many people end up taking them long term, despite the fact that little is known about how effective they are over the long haul. Prescription or over-the-counter medicines can have many problems, and while they can help in the short run, they nonetheless don't usually fix the underlying reasons for the type of sleep difficulties that many people have. Instead, some of the best longer-term solutions involve changes in a person's own behavior and sleep hygiene.

Stimulants

The influence of medications on the developing nervous system in young people may be even more complex than the influence of medications in older people. With that said, stimulants, such as medications containing amphetamine (e.g., Adderall) and Ritalin (methylphenidate), can substantially benefit children with attention deficit hyperactivity disorder (ADHD), a condition that can severely interfere with a child's function and school performance. Stimulants allow children to focus and pay attention, which helps with school performance and homework. These drugs can also help with social interactions. Like all drugs, they also have side effects, including nervousness, decreased appetite, sleep changes, and a slight decrease in the rate of a child's growth. Stimulants are also sometimes used to treat depression, although they are fourth- or fifth-line treatments, well behind the antidepressants described previously. Obviously, significant discussions should occur among the family, teachers, and health care team regarding this important category of drugs.

Stimulant-type drugs can also increase concentration in people without ADHD. Sometimes, college students without ADHD take these drugs to help them to study longer. This type of stimulant use has not been well studied, and we know little about the risk. It is possible, however, that these students may be at increased risk for abusing the drug recreationally for its pleasurable effects, given the history of similar abuse of other stimulants (e.g., cocaine and methamphetamine). Related to this, children and adolescents who are taking stimulants appropriately for ADHD may be approached by other students who want to buy the drugs for their own illicit use. Similarly, there is evidence that drug abusers can modify certain stimulants chemically to create drugs with even more powerful abuse potential. For these reasons, some psychiatrists prefer to use stimulant preparations that are less likely to be abused (e.g., slower-release preparations). Much more research is necessary to fully understand the benefits, risks, and misuse of these drugs.

Sometimes, as young people mature, they grow out of ADHD. For others, however, the symptoms continue throughout their lives. Adult-onset ADHD, on the other hand, is probably rare. People who have initial ADHD symptoms as adults should be carefully evaluated for other disorders, including substance abuse. Psychological tests that measure cognitive performance under controlled circumstances can be useful for determining the type of dysfunction. Otherwise, since there are no definitive tests for ADHD, caution should be used in prescribing ADHD medications in adults. Some adults with lifelong ADHD truly benefit from stimulants and don't abuse them. But other adults with recent onset of ADHD-like symptoms, especially individuals with a history of drug abuse and therefore an increased risk of abusing stimulants, should be evaluated carefully, with follow-up and re-evaluation as necessary, and alternative diagnoses and treatments should be considered.

An alternative to the stimulants in treating ADHD in both children and adults is Strattera (atomoxetine), which acts by blocking the uptake of the neurotransmitter norepinephrine. It has beneficial effects on concentration and attention, and its abuse potential appears to be less than that of the stimulants. In some ways, Strattera is like some antidepressant drugs that block norepinephrine uptake, but it doesn't appear to act as an antidepressant.

Medications for Drug Dependency Disorders

Medications can help persons with addictive disorders, but they are of limited usefulness unless they are combined with psychosocial interventions. Because addictive drugs can lead to long-lasting changes in the brain, long-term interventions may be necessary. In fact, certain abused drugs can result in such powerful addictions that these illnesses may be best viewed as chronic disorders requiring life-long treatment. We will briefly review medication strategies involved in the treatment of addiction to three drugs in particular: nicotine, alcohol, and opiates (specifically heroin).

Nicotine

As is well known, the addicting chemical in cigarettes is nicotine. There are two major medication strategies to help someone quit cigarettes. The first approach involves nicotine substitution, which is a means of providing nicotine via a safer delivery system than cigarettes. Some of these nicotine-delivery systems are available over the counter, such as nicotine patches, and others require a prescription. Nicotine substitution allows a person to continue receiving doses of nicotine while learning how to minimize and avoid behaviors that are associated with cigarette smoking. It is not just the nicotine that is addicting; the physical act of smoking, with the associated use of hands and the smell of cigarette smoke, and the various social settings where the person enjoys smoking all become associated with the addiction. Group therapy, individual therapy, or Internet-based interventions can be helpful to a person who is learning how to handle the cravings to smoke. As a person begins to learn to live without cigarettes, he or she can slowly decrease the nicotine dose. As any former smoker knows, it may take months or even years before the temptation to smoke diminishes. In some cases, it never goes away completely.

Among prescription nicotine substitutes is a medication called Chantix (varenicline), which works by stimulating certain nicotine receptors in the brain. It helps to prevent physical symptoms of nicotine withdrawal during the time when a person is dealing with the non-nicotine aspects of cigarette dependence. Eventually, as a person gets better control over the smoking habit, the dose of this medication is decreased and eventually stopped. Recent reports suggesting that Chantix has serious side effects in some individuals, including agitation, depression, and suicidal ideas, may limit the use of this medication, however.

A different type of medication used to help a person quit cigarettes is Wellbutrin (bupropion), an antidepressant medication discussed previously. Bupropion is also marketed under the name Zyban for its use in smoking cessation (note that this is a marketing strategy and that the active ingredient in Wellbutrin and Zyban is actually the same). Although we don't fully understand how bupropion works, it appears to stimulate the brain's reward systems and, in so doing, can partially substitute for the rewarding effects of cigarettes and decrease the desire to smoke. This mechanism, therefore, is quite different than nicotine substitution. But can the two approaches work well together? At the current time, some data suggest that nicotine-directed treatments together with bupropion may have additive effectiveness; that is, the two approaches may be more effective when used in combination than either alone. Similarly, pairing nicotine patches with other forms of nicotine-delivery systems, such as nicotine gum, may have additive effects as well. Presently, Chantix does not appear to have additive effects with other pharmacologic treatments. Also, it is worth re-emphasizing that medication treatments for smoking cessation are much more effective when coupled with group therapy or other types of psychological interventions. The Public Health Services' publication, "Treating Tobacco Use and Dependence: 2008 Update," is a valuable resource on this topic.

Alcohol

The first step in treating alcohol dependence is to help the patient stop drinking in a manner that avoids dangerous and potentially life-threatening withdrawal symptoms. This step may take a week or two. During this time, careful medical observation may be needed, together with a medicine that can partially substitute for alcohol. A benzodiazepine such as Valium (diazepam), Librium (chlordiazepoxide), or Ativan (lorazepam) can be helpful in preventing severe medical problems that can arise from the sudden cessation of drinking. Once a person is safely off alcohol, the Valium-like drug can be tapered and stopped.

Sustained psychosocial support is frequently necessary to enable people to successfully overcome their addiction to alcohol. Several counseling approaches may help a person develop the coping mechanisms necessary to resist the very strong desire to return to drinking. One of these, called "motivational interviewing," seems particularly useful. This is a form of therapist–patient interaction that focuses on dealing with the patient's awareness of the problem and its consequences while helping, in a nonjudgmental and nonconfrontational fashion, to increase the patient's desire to change.

In addition, some medications can help decrease the craving for alcohol and the frequency and severity of relapses. One of these drugs is Revia (naltrexone), which works by blocking certain opiate receptors in the brain. This opiate system influences the same brain reward system that is influenced by alcohol. By decreasing the influence of the opiate system, Revia helps to diminish the desire for alcohol. Another drug called Campral (acamprosate) also helps to decrease the attractiveness of alcohol. The exact mechanism of this agent is unknown, although it may influence brain transmitter systems—GABA and glutamate in particular—that are also acted upon by alcohol. Neither Revia nor Campral are miracle drugs. They can only assist a motivated person who is also undergoing psychosocial treatment to maintain sobriety.

A totally different medication approach to achieving sobriety is offered by a drug called Antabuse (disulfiram), the oldest of the available medication treatments for alcoholism. This drug interferes with the way the body chemically handles alcohol. In the process, a toxic substance accumulates in the body whenever a person drinks alcohol. This toxic byproduct of alcohol causes a person to become extremely nauseated. The problem with this drug is that the side effects are so unpleasant that it takes a very motivated person to continue treatment, and it may be this motivation and not the drug itself that produces the benefits.

Opiates

Opiate dependence can involve illegal substances, such as heroin, or prescription pain medications, such as Oxycontin (oxycodone). Legal or illegal, these drugs influence similar brain systems. The effects of opiates vary depending on the route of administration. Snorting heroin through the nose has a more powerfully addicting effect than taking a tablet of Oxycontin orally; shooting heroin intravenously has an even more powerful effect, including a "rush" that has a pleasurable feeling described as akin to an orgasm. Regardless of the route of administration, however, each of these agents can eventually become very habit forming. Heroin is among the most dangerous drugs in terms of its potential for addiction. In fact, heroin can have such strong effects on the brain that they may be very hard to reverse completely.

One medication strategy to treat heroin addiction involves substituting a longer-lasting but gentler opiate for heroin. One such substitute is methadone, and its use as a maintenance treatment decreases the craving for other opiates such as heroin and thereby diminishes the drug-seeking behaviors that dominate an addict's life. Rather than spending their lives preoccupied with finding the next heroin fix or procuring the money to buy it, people on methadone are able to participate in normal activities of daily living. Methadone stays in the body long enough that it needs to be taken only once a day. A person can take methadone for years and function well. However, it is still a powerful and addicting medication. Because of this, only specially licensed centers are allowed to offer methadone maintenance treatment. Some patients may eventually try to slowly taper off of the methadone. Others find they cannot get by without it. They come to view their condition as a chronic illness requiring chronic treatment.

Recently, another agent called buprenorphine has been approved for treatment of opiate addiction. This agent also has opiate properties, but it is less strong than heroin. Buprenorphine helps to block the effect of heroin and, similar to methadone, can help a person focus on activities of daily living, free of the dominant need to get high from heroin. A medication called Suboxone contains buprenorphine together with naloxone. Naloxone blocks opiate receptors in the brain and would lead to an immediate and very painful opiate withdrawal if absorbed into the bloodstream. For this reason, Suboxone is taken orally as a pill that is placed under the tongue and allowed to dissolve. Taken this way, the naloxone in the Suboxone does not get absorbed and hence does not block the action of the buprenorphine and lead to withdrawal. However, if a person were to inject the Suboxone in order to try to get high from the buprenorphine, the naloxone component would block the effects of buprenorphine and lead to a major opiate withdrawal. Ideally, once a person has been on Suboxone for an extended period of time, he or she might try to taper and perhaps eventually stop the medication. Since there is less risk of abuse of Suboxone than of methadone, a person is not required to attend a specially licensed clinic to obtain this medication. Rather, a physician who has taken special training in the proper use of Suboxone is eligible to prescribe it in limited quantities.

Over recent years, the brain systems involved in drug addiction have become much better understood. As scientists learn how to reverse the changes caused by these drugs, major advances in the treatment of the addiction disorders are likely to occur.

Over-the-Counter Medications or Herbal Remedies for Psychiatric Disorders

There are thousands of herbal remedies and over-the-counter products. While it is beyond our scope to review the various classes of such products that claim to benefit people with psychiatric symptoms, we would emphasize the following points:

- These products may contain active ingredients that can influence your body and your brain; many of the effects can be harmful.

- These products are drugs and may interact with other over-the-counter products or with prescribed medications.

- Although some data exist suggesting that some products may work for certain disorders, we don't have reliable and valid studies documenting the effectiveness of most of these products. There is a branch of the National Institutes of Health (NIH) that has ongoing studies examining some of the more promising over-the-counter products.

- Just because a product is available without a doctor's prescription does not mean it is safe.

- Just because a product is "natural" does not mean it is safe. For example, snake venom is a natural substance; so is arsenic.

- Be skeptical about claims made about these products; hucksters exist all over our planet and these remedies are a big business.

- It is important to let your health care team know if you are using a particular product.

With those cautions, we would make several concluding comments. Some people try various herbal products and find that they are beneficial. Others get into trouble with side effects or drug interactions. There are risks involved with many of these substances. Unfortunately, it is difficult and sometimes impossible to make rational decisions regarding a large number of these products because they simply have not been studied in sufficient detail. In the absence of sound data coming from well-done clinical trials, we would recommend extreme caution in using any of these products.

Take-Home Messages

- There is an array of medication approaches available for treating psychiatric disorders. All can produce significant benefits but are also associated with side effects. The choice of treatment for any patient is always made in collaboration between the doctor and the patient and takes into account a careful analysis of the risk-benefit ratio. As is true of most of medicine, the treatments in psychiatry can be highly effective, but they are not cures.

- Medications have become mainstays for managing most serious psychiatric disorders. This does not minimize the importance of psychotherapy and social interventions, but rather it reflects the overall effectiveness and ease of use of the medications. Despite this, medications are far from perfect and don't help every patient.

All medications have side effects. This is true for all medications in all branches of medicine.

- By becoming knowledgeable about psychiatric medications—about both their effects and their side effects—patients and their families become better-informed consumers and collaborators in the treatment process.

- Over-the-counter drugs and herbal treatments are big businesses in the United States. The scientific basis for many of these treatments is extremely limited. Patients should be aware of this and make sure that their doctors know about *all* medications, prescription and otherwise, that they are taking. This is the only way physicians are able to assess the side effects and benefits of other treatments.

··· nine ···

Psychotherapies and Lifestyle Interventions

Psychiatrists and mental health professionals use a variety of methods to treat patients with psychiatric disorders. In the previous chapter, we discussed psychotropic medications. In the next chapter, we will discuss brain stimulation methods, such as electroconvulsive therapy. These are not the only weapons available, and other forms of treatment, including various forms of talk therapy (psychotherapy) and lifestyle interventions, can be extremely valuable in achieving optimal outcomes. An important principle to remember is that no one treatment is appropriate for all patients; effective care must be tailored to the needs of the individual patient. As we have noted previously, there are no cures for psychiatric disorders. However, there is considerable hope and opportunity for improvement in the outcome of these disorders, including by mechanisms through which patients can alter their own thinking and lifestyle to gain control over their symptoms. In this sense, psychiatric care is a bit like rehabilitative medicine where physicians work with a team of other health care providers to help patients with chronic and at times debilitating illnesses function at the highest level possible. A good portion of rehabilitative care is directed toward controlling symptoms and helping patients manage their lives as independently as they can. In our opinion, this is the essence of what psychological and lifestyle interventions in psychiatry are all about. The interaction between patients and their treatment providers is largely geared toward educating patients (and their families) about the illnesses—helping them to understand and minimize symptoms and complications—and working on their relationships, employment, and overall function.

The Importance of Human Interactions

Humans are inherently social animals and generally benefit from social contacts. Meaningful social interactions have helped us to survive as a species and are important for our survival as individuals. Thus, it should not be surprising that meaningful dialogues with mental health professionals can benefit people with psychiatric illnesses. As emphasized throughout this book, the benefits of this type of interaction are not unique to psychiatry, and there is considerable evidence that patients with any medical disorder benefit from concerned and consistent interactions with their health care providers. Medications prescribed without careful follow-up do not work as well as medications prescribed in the setting of frequent and compassionate follow-up. Excellent medical care requires the demonstrated interest and concern of the doctor and the health care team. When patients and families deal with a team they know, they develop trust and are more likely to comply with treatment recommendations.

Even with devastating neurodegenerative disorders like Alzheimer's disease, participants in clinical trials who are treated with placebo medication ("sugar pills") tend to improve during the first weeks of study. Why does this happen even in an illness like Alzheimer's disease? It is likely that attention from families, nurses, study personnel, and doctors helps people feel better such that they perform better on the different types of testing involved in the study. Other studies that compare a group receiving medication plus usual medical care with a group receiving medication plus more extensive, comprehensive medical follow-up demonstrate that participants in the more comprehensive follow-up group tend to respond better to treatment. This more intensive treatment isn't really anything out of the ordinary; it is just good medical care. Human interaction at the level of a caring treatment team can make a huge difference in clinical outcome. The corollary to this point is that patients and their families must believe that the treatment team is listening and communicating with them. If this is not the case, it may be appropriate to seek treatment elsewhere.

Another type of potentially helpful human interaction involves support groups. People feel better when they communicate with others who face the same challenges. There is something comforting about being able to share thoughts and emotions with those who are experiencing similar issues. Support groups exist for people with just about any illness, including cancer, Alzheimer's disease, depression, schizophrenia, and substance abuse, although each group may differ from others in the type of approach it takes among its members. For substance abuse support groups, for example, the approach will likely differ depending on the drug of abuse. Groups dealing with nicotine addiction may use different approaches than groups that help people maintain recovery from alcohol or narcotics. There is something very human about the fact that peer support helps our brains retrain and perhaps even reverse the biological changes that addicting drugs cause.

Other forms of interpersonal interactions are designed to help patients with various aspects of their lives. This help may include professional counseling about interpersonal relationships (marital or couples therapy); training related to job skills, financial planning, and debt repayment; and in severe cases, assistance with disability planning and Social Security. Many of these areas fall outside the expertise of psychiatrists and involve other members of the mental health team, particularly professionals trained in social work and specific counseling services. All of these areas can be extremely important in the rehabilitative process of treating mental illnesses.

Education is a significant component of all of the aforementioned forms of treatment. People come to their physicians with various levels of knowledge about psychiatric illness; some of it is accurate, and some of it is just plain wrong. One of the psychiatrist's major roles is to help people understand the nature of their disorder and the expectations they should have about its treatment and outcome. Accurate information is empowering. The more that patients and families know about the disorder that has engulfed their lives, the more they can effectively participate as part of the treatment team.

Specific Psychotherapies

In addition to the very important interactions that patients have with health care teams and support groups, there are specific forms of psychological treatments that may be useful in certain disorders. These psychotherapies are typically based on one-on-one interactions with a therapist or, in some cases, on group interactions with a therapist. The group psychotherapies can be viewed as extensions of the support group concept, although they are based on more formal principles of psychotherapy. Psychotherapies can vary widely in how they are conducted. Similarly, there is wide variability in the expertise and skill of psychotherapists. Some forms of psychotherapy are administered in highly structured formats, while others are much less formal. By "structured" we mean forms of therapy that follow protocols developed by experts in the field; these protocols may deal with how often sessions are held, how questions are asked and answered, and whether homework assignments are used to assist patients outside the individual sessions. Increasingly, the structured therapies are being studied in rigorous clinical trials, and available evidence suggests that they are more effective than less structured therapies.

How psychotherapies help patients with psychiatric disorders is also an area of active research. Some psychotherapies may work by influencing specific areas of the brain, and different psychotherapies may influence different brain regions. For instance, some people fear heights and/or bridges. By exposing such a person to controlled but increasing intensities of fear-inducing stimuli related to the specific phobia, the person is gradually desensitized to the emotional and cognitive responses evoked by these stimuli. This approach appears to work by retraining certain regions of the brain involved with emotions, but these regions may differ from those that are influenced by some of the other therapies to be discussed shortly.

This "desensitization" treatment is part of a general class called "behavioral therapy," and a key component of this kind of therapy is to combine exposure to bothersome activities or thoughts with exercises that help the patient remain calm and in control. These exercises typically involve forms of "relaxation therapy" in which patients are taught techniques that help them to diminish their cognitive, emotional, and physical responses to stress. Some therapists use measurements of muscle tension, skin response, heart rate, breathing rate, or other bodily measurements to help patients deal with specific symptoms and to determine whether the relaxation techniques are having the desired effects. While such "biofeedback" can be useful under some circumstances, its role in the treatment of many stress-related conditions is not clear cut. Importantly, however, stress management in some form is a key component of most forms of psychotherapy. For some individuals, help with controlling their anger via cognitive and behavioral approaches is also critical in helping them learn to deal more effectively with symptoms or problems.

Cognitive Behavioral Therapy

The structured psychotherapy that has received the most systematic study and has the best overall track record is cognitive behavioral therapy (CBT). CBT was developed by psychiatrist Aaron Beck and colleagues at the University of Pennsylvania. It involves helping patients understand that thoughts and feelings are interrelated and that the way people think has a big effect on their mood and emotions. The basic principle of CBT is that if people can retrain their thinking through rational examination of their thoughts and assumptions, they can help control their symptoms. Learning to avoid unhealthy and automatic patterns of thinking is part of the process. When patients come to negative conclusions about life events or issues, they are encouraged to reconsider their conclusions and to challenge the assumptions that led to those conclusions. CBT combines behavioral techniques with teaching people to analyze their responses to certain situations logically. During the early phases of treatment, the behavioral component of CBT can be particularly important in helping patients to increase their activity levels and improve their self-reliance. As part of both the cognitive and behavioral components of CBT, therapists assign homework designed to help patients work on aspects of therapy covered during individual sessions. Formal CBT usually involves a series of sessions held once or twice per week over a defined period of time. Follow-up sessions are held at varying intervals to reinforce the benefits of the more intensive initial sessions. How long therapy continues may be defined at the outset of therapy or decided by mutual agreement between the patient and therapist as treatment progresses.

CBT can be very helpful for some disorders but is not as useful for other conditions. For example, studies have shown that CBT is useful in treating mild to moderate forms of major depression. However, it is less effective against severe psychotic depressions, particularly during the phase when patients are experiencing delusions and hallucinations. Interestingly, CBT may be helpful for some problems that have psychiatric overtones but are not considered to be primary psychiatric disorders. These include some forms of chronic insomnia and perhaps chronic pain. CBT may also be useful for diminishing the relapse potential in patients with depression or anxiety disorders after remission of a current episode. This latter aspect may be one of the most important facets of this type of therapy.

Several other therapies also employ cognitive and behavioral techniques. These include dialectical behavioral therapy (DBT), which is used in patients with borderline personality disorder and recurrent suicidal behaviors, and the cognitive behavioral analysis system of psychotherapy (CBASP), which is used for treating some chronic depressions. DBT was developed by psychologist Marsha Linehan and focuses heavily on correcting maladaptive patterns of behavior (including recurrent self-injury), but it also uses techniques akin to those used in CBT with a strong effort directed at developing problem-solving skills. DBT therapists help patients deal nonjudgmentally with difficulties in regulating their emotions, handling distress, and interacting with other people. CBASP aims to help patients learn appropriate and mature coping skills and to take charge of their own lives while overcoming maladaptive responses learned from adverse early life experiences. DBT and CBASP are potentially important therapies that extend the basic principles of CBT, and studies examining their effectiveness are in progress. At present, CBT remains the standard against which these other therapies are generally compared.

Interpersonal Therapy

Interpersonal therapy (IPT) is a form of psychotherapy that focuses on a patient's current relationships and interpersonal problems. IPT is a time-limited treatment and is based on the idea that problems in relationships result in a great deal of stress. Therefore, helping patients confront these problems can go a long way toward improving mood and anxiety symptoms. IPT has been studied in a number of well-designed clinical trials, and like CBT, it has a favorable track record in treating mild to moderately severe major depression.

IPT is a "here and now" type of treatment. The sessions are targeted toward current, not past, problems in relationships and address how interpersonal problems are affecting the patient and others. The therapist plays an active but nonjudgmental role in helping individuals to understand how their current interpersonal problems are affecting their symptoms and function. Effort is directed toward one or two problem areas that the patient and therapist agree are of importance (e.g., marital discord or problems at work). The emphasis is not as much on negative and automatic thinking as in CBT, but rather on distortions in how the patient perceives and responds to current relationships.

Insight-Oriented Psychotherapies

Some psychotherapies are aimed at helping patients gain insight into the factors that influence their thinking and behavior. In effect, this is what the cognitive part of CBT is about. Another type of psychotherapy known as insight-oriented or psychodynamic therapy focuses specifically on the goal of helping individuals understand why they think and behave the way they do. Psychodynamic psychotherapy grew out of the psychoanalytic approach to psychiatric disorders and traces its roots back to Sigmund Freud. At one time, this was the dominant approach to psychotherapy in the United States and is the form of psychotherapy that many patients associate with psychiatry. Today, psychodynamic therapy is only one of several approaches that are commonly used. Insight-oriented therapy typically involves approximately one-hour sessions one or more times a week for several months or years. During this therapy, patients explore how their past may be influencing the present. Psychodynamic therapists place significant emphasis on understanding the unconscious mental processes that contribute to a patient's behavior and thinking, and on understanding the psychological defense mechanisms that a patient uses to function. The goal of understanding these issues is to develop healthier and more mature ways of thinking about and dealing with the world.

Some insight-oriented therapies can be time-limited and targeted to specific situations; other therapies can be extended. The extended approaches are costly, and data indicating their benefit have been difficult to generate. Presently, the evidence supporting psychodynamic therapy lags behind evidence supporting CBT, behavioral therapy, and IPT. Nevertheless, some people are likely to derive significant benefit from the insights they gain from psychodynamic approaches.

A potentially important development has been the generation of structured forms of insight-oriented therapy. An example is mentalization-based therapy for use in the treatment of patients with borderline personality disorder. "Mentalization" is an important concept that reflects the ability of our minds (brains) to recognize our own mental states and to recognize that others have minds that are different from ours. In this form of therapy, patients are helped to understand their own changing states of mind and to develop alternative views of themselves and others. The therapy shares principles with "transference-focused" forms of psychotherapy. Transference is a psychodynamic concept that refers to the idea that how we respond currently to people in our lives (particularly authority figures like psychotherapists) reflects unconscious attributions developed toward others early in life. Learning to deal with these unconscious attributions can help patients understand their own current behavior and thinking. While still in development, these forms of insight-oriented therapy have shown promise in the management of some personality disorders; if this continues to hold true, it could be a useful advance for the field.

Supportive and Other Psychotherapies

Another form of psychotherapy that most patients are likely to encounter during their routine psychiatric care goes under the general heading of "supportive psychotherapy." This form of treatment strives to identify and build on a person's current strengths, using those strengths to help the individual better cope with specific situations and challenges. Most mental health practitioners use some form of supportive therapy and may include elements derived from CBT, IPT, and insight-oriented therapy, among others. The term *supportive psychotherapy* is sometimes used rather loosely to mean nonspecific treatment. In fact, supportive approaches utilize specific psychotherapy techniques and can be extremely beneficial to patients and their families.

Many forms of psychotherapy have come and gone. Logotherapy, gestalt therapy, and transactional analysis come to mind as examples. Other therapies are in various stages of development. One criticism of some of the current psychotherapies is that they overly focus on psychiatric symptoms and negative thinking. In response to this perceived deficit, there are some efforts to develop well being-based approaches that emphasize positive emotions, engagement with others, and life meaning. One example is "positive psychotherapy," which is being developed by psychologist Martin Seligman and colleagues.

Increasingly, psychotherapies are being rigorously studied in terms of their effectiveness. As the future evolves, evidence-based psychotherapies—that is, those with well-designed studies to support their effectiveness—will become the standard used to judge which therapies are offered to patients and reimbursed by third-party payers.

The Importance of the Therapist

In many cases, the benefits of a particular therapy appear to depend less on the specific techniques used than on the personal characteristics of therapists themselves—their warmth, empathy, genuineness, and understanding as perceived by the patient. These features, like training, vary widely among therapists, and patients are advised to use their judgment to determine whether a therapist's interpersonal style is right for them. Just as there is no one treatment that is right for all patients, no one therapist or physician is right for all patients.

It is also important to realize that psychotherapies are powerful techniques that can influence and change the brain. (When we learn anything, there are changes in our brains.) The idea that psychotherapies just involve talking and therefore can't have side effects is wrong. Psychotherapies can have tremendous benefits, but they also can have risks. For example, in the recent past, some well-meaning, but scientifically naive therapists encouraged highly suggestible patients to develop false memories about being abused earlier in life, and these false memories led to a great deal of personal and interpersonal strife. The therapies we have emphasized in this chapter are among the best validated in psychiatry and psychology. By "validated" we mean that they have been studied in rigorous and well-designed clinical trials. There are a number of other therapies used to treat psychiatric disorders that have limited validation and, in some cases, no or limited basis in any science. Examples from the recent past include therapies that used hypnosis to help recover "repressed" memories and therapies to help uncover lost (or multiple) personalities. Many of these fall under the rubric of pseudoscience and are more harmful than helpful. It can be extremely difficult for patients to know what constitutes a validated therapy. Our descriptions are a brief introduction to the topic and patients are encouraged to consult local chapters of the American Psychiatric Association or American Psychological Association for further guidance.

We would also emphasize that an effective therapist can become a powerful figure in a patient's life, and this, too, can have consequences. Sometimes, therapists may be too forceful in encouraging major life changes at inappropriate times. Such poorly timed life changes can be harmful. Words and human interactions can have powerful effects, and patients must remain aware of this fact.

The Role of Psychiatrists in Psychotherapy

Psychiatrists often develop treatment plans that utilize medications and various psychotherapeutic techniques. Does this mean that a psychiatrist will personally administer a complete course of a specific form of structured psychotherapy? This varies from psychiatrist to psychiatrist but is often not the case. More often, psychiatrists use techniques based on a variety of therapeutic approaches combined with patient education. Treatment that combines medications with the use of these techniques in several follow-up visits is frequently sufficient to help a person begin to feel much better. If it appears that a patient would benefit from a longer or more structured program of a specific formal psychotherapy (e.g., CBT), the psychiatrist may refer the person to a therapist trained in that particular technique. It is less common today for psychiatrists to provide long-term, intensive therapies themselves. When such a team approach is used, it is always in a patient's best interest for the various members of the health care team (both physical and mental health teams) to stay in fairly close contact. Again, the patient must know who the point person is and how information among members of the treatment team is being coordinated.

Practices vary greatly in terms of which members of the mental health team participate in various aspects of treatment. Sometimes, patients' insurance companies have preferences in this regard as well. Managed care companies frequently encourage psychiatrists to restrict their roles to diagnosis and biologic treatments. These third-party payers prefer that longer-term courses of psychotherapy be administered by therapists who are less expensive than psychiatrists. Such therapists include psychologists, social workers, and counselors with various levels of professional training.

Because of the shortage in the number of psychiatrists, it is imperative that teams of mental health professionals are used in order to reach the large number of patients needing mental health services. Collaborative models have been developed for recognizing and treating depression in the primary care setting. These models integrate the expertise of various mental health professionals as needed. For example, patients are screened for depression in a primary care setting, utilizing simple assessment tools. If a patient is assessed as having clinically significant depressive symptoms, the primary care team initiates treatment that may include an antidepressant coupled with close follow-up and pragmatic counseling. If symptoms improve, the treatment plan is continued. If symptoms become worse, or if improvement doesn't occur over a reasonable amount of time, specialized counselors or psychiatrists may become more directly involved in the patient's care. These models can utilize efficient, informal consultations between the primary care team and psychiatrists and, depending on the patient's response to treatment, face-to-face meetings between the psychiatrist and the patient.

Lifestyle Changes and Psychiatry

We have briefly reviewed many of the biologic and psychotherapeutic approaches utilized by psychiatrists and other mental health providers to treat psychiatric disorders. In addition to these treatments, it is becoming increasingly apparent that patients can do a lot to help themselves, and this may be one of the most important factors in determining lasting improvements. We are learning that many behaviors that have been popularly labeled as "heart healthy" are likely to be "brain healthy" as well. These behaviors include controlling blood pressure, lowering high cholesterol, minimizing alcohol use, and avoiding cigarettes. Watching one's weight and paying attention to eating a balanced diet can also be helpful for both physical and mental health. We sometimes refer to the adoption of these healthy behaviors as "TLC"— "therapeutic lifestyle changes."

Animal research strongly suggests that caloric restriction in adult life is a major factor in increased and healthy longevity. In addition, certain dietary components are likely to have important health benefits. For example, the omega-3 fatty acids found in certain fish such as salmon are likely to be beneficial to our hearts and possibly our brains. It has become evident that changes in modern western diets over the last several hundred years have significantly altered the ratio of omega-3 fatty acids to omega-6 fatty acids (found in unsaturated vegetable oils) that people consume. This change may result in significant health consequences, including increased risk of heart attacks and possibly several mental disorders. We are, however, only just beginning to understand the long-term effects of dietary changes on the physical and mental health of humans. The omega-3 fish oil story is just beginning to be systematically studied, and we will learn much more about the psychiatric effects of rebalancing this nutrient in the future.

Other much-ballyhooed nutrients, however, may not be so promising. As with the over-the-counter remedies for psychiatric disorders that we mentioned in the previous chapter, a large industry related to dietary "health" supplements now exists. Advocates make dramatic claims about the health benefits of these nutrients, and advertisements are found everywhere claiming that certain supplements can help with weight loss, sexual performance, strength, arthritis, etc. Some of these supplements may do no harm and may, in fact, prove to be beneficial. Others may be quite harmful. Again, until well-designed and reproducible studies demonstrate the benefits of specific supplements, it is best to be cautious before accepting health claims from the companies that produce these products and the health care providers who hawk them. And as always, your health care team needs to know about any dietary supplements you are taking or dietary changes you are making.

Many Americans suffer from obesity, and the obesity epidemic is now rampant in our youth. Obesity contributes to numerous health problems, including chronic illnesses like diabetes, coronary heart disease, and sleep problems. It likely has major mental health consequences as well. Depression, for instance, is extremely common in people with diabetes and in those suffering from coronary heart disease. Moreover, Americans generally pay little attention to physical activity and exercise, and they potentially face adverse health consequences as a result. There is increasing evidence that exercise is associated with good health, with the direct effects of exercise likely leading to changes that affect many of our bodily systems, including the brain. In fact, studies are demonstrating that routine exercise and weight reduction correlate with longevity and decreased prevalence of certain medical and psychiatric disorders.

Finally, many experts are starting to believe that healthy play during childhood is important for strong emotional development. Experts in animal behaviors, such as Jaak Panksepp, have demonstrated the importance of interactive play in the social development of a wide variety of animals. Positive social interactions early in life probably help the developing brain become better able to handle interactions and stresses later in life. Importantly, the play that appears to be the most beneficial is physical play combining exercise and enjoyment. Socially isolated play, including Internet surfing and watching video games, does not appear to carry the same benefits. For adults, various forms of interactive play are likely to be equally important as a means of physical activity and stress reduction. The old adage about "all work and no play" is true.

A key point in this discussion is that heart- and brain-healthy behaviors are under the control of patients—not their doctors. Doctors can't make patients do these things. But when patients pay attention to diet, weight, sleep hygiene, and exercise, there are likely to be benefits for multiple aspects of their lives. These interventions also cost very little, and their benefit-risk ratio is potentially very large. We would emphasize, however, that patients should implement these suggestions in collaboration with their physicians and increase their activity gradually depending on tolerance.

In this chapter, we have outlined a variety of approaches that psychiatrists and other mental health professionals use in managing psychiatric disorders. A theme that we hope is evident in this discussion is that there is nothing magical about psychotherapy, social interventions, and lifestyle changes. These approaches are largely built on principles of rehabilitative medicine and involve a lot of common sense. Some therapists and other professionals will likely disagree with these concepts, but we would argue strongly that therapy is all about common sense. In fact, we would state that if an approach used by a therapist doesn't make sense to the patient, then the patient should perhaps consider finding another therapist. Seemingly mystical or unrealistic explanations about illnesses and behavior may say more about the therapist than about the disorder being treated.

Take-Home Messages

- Human interaction at the level of a caring treatment team can make a huge difference in clinical outcome. When patients and families deal with a mental health team they know, they develop trust and are more likely to comply with and respond positively to treatment recommendations.

- Humans are social animals. People tend to benefit from group support when facing any serious illness. This is the essence of group therapies and support groups.

- There are specific forms of psychological therapies that may be helpful for specific conditions. These therapies may help diminish the risk of relapse in a number of disorders, including major depression.

- Like all treatments in medicine, psychotherapies have both potential risks and potential benefits. There is a tendency on the part of professionals to minimize the risks, but these can be significant, as in the "recovered memory" fiasco.

- Lifestyle changes that are heart healthy are also likely to be brain healthy. Diet and exercise are not only good for the heart, but they can also help in the management of a variety of mental disorders. Patients can control these aspects of their care.

- It appears likely that certain forms of play during childhood and even adulthood assist in the development and maintenance of interactive skills and can benefit mental health.

- Psychotherapy is not magic. The approaches and explanations provided by therapists should be based in common sense and make sense to the patient. Having said that, the benefits of psychotherapy can be "magical" in helping patients deal with their symptoms and life circumstances. Psychotherapy is part of all good psychiatric care.

ten

Brain Stimulation Methods

The use of brain stimulation methods to treat psychiatric disorders has a long history, antedating the modern psychopharmacology era by several decades. These treatments are among the most invasive used in psychiatry. By "invasive" we mean that these treatments are medical procedures. They can have dramatically beneficial effects but carry risks of significant side effects. The best-known and most-studied brain stimulation method is electroconvulsive therapy (ECT), a treatment that has been used in psychiatry since the 1930s. Over the past decade or so, several other methods have been investigated, and these treatments are in various stages of development for potential clinical use. These latter treatments include vagus nerve stimulation, repetitive transcranial magnetic stimulation, and deep brain stimulation. We will discuss each of these methods in this chapter and try to clarify their potential in the management of psychiatric disorders.

Electroconvulsive Therapy

ECT is a procedure that is shrouded in more mystique and misunderstanding than perhaps any other treatment in medicine. Images of "shock therapy" from the movie *One Flew Over the Cuckoo's Nest* represent many people's misconceptions about how ECT is done and why it is used. The use of electrical stimulation for therapeutic purposes grew out of work in the early 20th century in which chemically induced seizures were found to have benefits for patients with psychotic disorders. The rationale was based on the incorrect idea that seizures and psychosis are incompatible. Early observations suggested that when patients had both epilepsy and psychosis, the psychosis seemed to decrease in severity when the seizures were more frequent and to worsen when the seizures were less frequent. Initial attempts to implement "convulsant treatments" used chemicals or gasses to induce seizures, but these were replaced in the 1930s by electrical stimulation, which proved more effective than drugs in controlling the induced seizures. Over the years, the technique for administering ECT has improved greatly, and today, despite advances in psychopharmacology, it remains the most effective treatment known for certain disorders.

ECT is most commonly used to treat major depression, particularly when the depression is severe and associated with psychosis, marked suicidal behavior, or the inability to feed or care for oneself. It also is effective for acute psychotic symptoms (delusions, hallucinations, and severe agitation) almost regardless of cause (e.g., schizophrenia, mood disorders including mania, or even medical conditions associated with psychosis). ECT is not effective for the chronic symptoms of schizophrenia, such as social withdrawal and cognitive dysfunction, and it is not helpful for treating personality disorders, somatization disorder, alcohol or drug abuse, and most anxiety disorders; however, even in these disorders, ECT can be useful when severe depression also is present. Because of the effectiveness of medications and psychotherapy and because of the side effects and social stigma associated with ECT, the procedure is usually a second- or third-line treatment, except in cases where patients have severe and life-threatening symptoms. In these latter cases, ECT can be lifesaving. ECT also plays an important role in the treatment of individuals who have failed to respond to prior treatment with psychiatric medications.

As a medical procedure, ECT is usually administered with written informed consent from the patient, although most jurisdictions allow the use of involuntary ECT in severe cases following local legal review. The procedure for obtaining permission for involuntary ECT is much like that for involuntary hospitalization described earlier in this book. Involuntary ECT is utilized only after an impartial judge is convinced during a legal hearing that other methods of treatment for a severe, life-threatening psychiatric condition have been exhausted or that the risks of not proceeding with ECT are too high.

As practiced today, ECT is always given under general anesthesia with muscle-relaxing drugs that are administered by injection through a vein (usually in the arm). Patients are thus not awake during the procedure and move very little during it because of the muscle relaxant. For these reasons, the treatment is done under highly controlled conditions involving a psychiatrist, an anesthesia provider, nurses, and technicians.

An actual ECT treatment takes about 15 minutes from start to finish, although recovery from the procedure can take another 45 to 60 minutes. Because one treatment is not sufficient to produce substantial clinical benefit, ECT is always given as a course of multiple treatments over a period of time. Courses of ECT vary, but typically a total of 8 to 12 treatments are administered at a rate of 2 or 3 individual treatments per week. ECT can be administered to patients on an in- or outpatient basis. Two forms of ECT are typically used: bilateral ECT (in which both sides of the head are stimulated) or unilateral ECT (in which only the nondominant [nonlanguage] side of the head is stimulated; this is almost always the right side). Both forms of ECT can be highly effective, but unilateral nondominant-hemisphere ECT causes much less memory loss and confusion compared to bilateral ECT. In turn, unilateral ECT is more difficult to administer and requires expertise in the selection of electrical doses.

The goal of ECT is to get symptoms of the psychiatric disorder into remission. Remission means having few or no remaining symptoms. Like all other treatments in psychiatry, ECT does not cure the underlying disorder. Thus, following a successful course of ECT, patients can expect to be treated with medications to help keep their disorder in remission. In cases where medications have been unsuccessful in maintaining remission of symptoms, ECT itself can be used as a maintenance treatment on an outpatient basis. When used for maintenance treatment, ECT is administered on a variable schedule, typically ranging from once a week to once a month (or less) depending on how the patient is doing and how well he or she tolerates the side effects of the procedure. Importantly, many cases that are said to be "ECT failures" actually reflect the failure of maintenance treatment and are not a failure of the initial course of ECT. But without effective maintenance treatment with medications, psychotherapy, or ECT, the risk of relapse is very high. The rate of relapse is greatest during the first several months after a successful course of treatment, so there is need for close follow-up with the treating psychiatrist during this period. This risk of relapse is not unique to ECT and is seen with medications as well. Thus, compliance with the maintenance phase of treatment is crucial if the best results are to be obtained.

Like all treatments in medicine, ECT has risks and side effects. Because the treatment is done under general anesthesia, involves electrical stimulation, and induces a generalized seizure in the brain, there is a small risk of death during the procedure. This risk is very low (something like the risk associated with childbirth), and ECT is actually a treatment of choice for some patients with severe medical and psychiatric disorders who cannot tolerate psychiatric medications. Heart problems (irregular heart rhythm or heart attack) are the biggest medical concerns with ECT, so particular attention is paid to cardiac risk factors when psychiatrists are considering patients for ECT. This may involve consultation with internists or cardiologists before starting treatment. Yet despite these risks, ECT can be safely used to treat a severe psychiatric disorder in patients with even severe heart disease.

Overall, an ECT treatment is a straightforward medical procedure, and most patients tolerate it very well. Some patients do, however, experience muscle soreness, headache, or nausea after a treatment; these side effects can be treated effectively with appropriate medications. But the biggest concern for most patients is memory loss and confusion. ECT does cause memory problems: Patients have difficulty recalling events that happen during the course of treatment (called "anterograde amnesia"), and some patients experience post-treatment difficulties with recalling things from earlier in their lives ("retrograde amnesia"). In general, these memory problems diminish with time after a course of ECT treatments is completed, but some patients do have persistent problems with recalling prior events. Importantly, the severe psychiatric disorders treated with ECT are also associated with cognitive impairment and memory difficulties, and in the case of major depression, many patients who have been treated successfully with ECT indicate that their memory is actually better after ECT than when they were severely depressed. That said, most advances in ECT technique, including the placement of stimulating electrodes, the electrical doses, the use of oxygen during the procedure, and the doses of anesthetics, have been tailored to diminish the memory loss from ECT to the extent possible.

One of the most frequently asked questions about ECT is "how does it work?" The truth is that we don't really know, just as we don't really know the mechanisms underlying psychiatric disorders in general. ECT produces numerous effects in the brain: Some of these effects mimic those of antidepressant drugs and are likely beneficial, and some cause side effects. Sorting this out is extremely difficult. What is known, based on numerous studies, is that ECT does not cause structural brain damage, contrary to the popular myth, held even among some psychiatrists, that it does. Also, it is known that the cognitive impairment from ECT is not part of the therapeutic effect. ECT does not produce benefits by making you forget your problems (another popular myth). Although ECT produces electrical seizures in the brain, it does not cause epilepsy. Interestingly, over a course of treatment, ECT actually has anticonvulsant effects, and in the past, it was sometimes used to treat patients who had forms of epilepsy that were difficult to control. Whether these anticonvulsant effects contribute to the therapeutic effects of ECT in psychiatric disorders is not certain. Current theories suggest that the beneficial effects of

ECT most likely involve effects on the neural circuitry underlying psychiatric disorders. Some evidence also indicates that ECT promotes the growth of new neurons in some regions of the brain, such as the dentate gyrus of the hippocampus. How and whether these "neurogenesis effects" relate to therapeutic effects is an area of active investigation in psychiatric neuroscience.

What is critical for patients and families to understand is that, despite its limitations, ECT does work. In fact, therapeutic responses to ECT can be among the most dramatic seen in psychiatry. Some of the sickest patients get tremendous and fairly rapid relief from their intense suffering. This treatment can be lifesaving.

Case Vignettes

In order to clarify the place of ECT as a therapeutic tool in psychiatry, we will describe two cases. While these are not real patients, they do represent the kind of cases referred to our ECT service.

Case I A 54-year-old man was admitted to the hospital after his wife discovered that he had purchased a gun and was planning to kill himself. He had also written a suicide note indicating his intentions. His wife convinced him to go with her to a local emergency room. In the emergency room, he described a three-month history of severe depressive symptoms that included low mood, inability to concentrate on his work, poor appetite with a 10-pound weight loss, poor sleep, and a strong desire to die. He was a successful businessman, and there were no ongoing stressors in his life. He was a social drinker but did not abuse alcohol or other drugs.

The physician in the emergency room consulted a psychiatrist and recommended psychiatric hospitalization. The patient reluctantly agreed and was started on antidepressant medication together with individual and group psychotherapy. After two weeks of treatment, his symptoms did not improve, and he still indicated a strong intent to take his own life. Although he felt that all attempts at treatment would fail, he consented to a trial of ECT. He received a total of eight right-unilateral treatments. Following the second treatment, his appetite started to improve and his suicidal ideas markedly diminished. He also started to interact with his family when they visited. Following the fourth treatment, he started to sleep through the night and regain interest in his business. He was able to watch a baseball game and enjoyed reading the newspaper. He noted some decrease in his memory for recent events, but did not report other side effects except for a mild headache following a treatment. The headaches improved with acetaminophen (Tylenol). Following his eighth treatment, his family reported that he was "like his old self." He had insight into his illness and was compliant with medications and counseling. He was discharged from the hospital on antidepressant medication and continued meeting weekly with his psychiatrist. After six months, his treatment consisted of an antidepressant medication and visits to his psychiatrist every three months.

He did well for the next five years and was active in both his business and social life. Then, he started to worry a great deal about work and developed sleep problems; he woke up in the middle of the night and was not able to get back to sleep. His psychiatrist increased the frequency of outpatient visits and increased the dose of his antidepressant. The symptoms worsened. The patient denied that the depression had reached the level where he was actively considering suicide. He participated in intensive outpatient management that included cognitive behavioral therapy and trials of different antidepressants at appropriate doses. Unfortunately, despite this aggressive treatment, suicidal thoughts returned suddenly. He attempted to kill himself by hanging, but the rope snapped. His wife heard him fall and brought him to the hospital. Because of his earlier response to ECT, he consented to a course of ECT. He once again responded well to this treatment and experienced complete remission of his symptoms after ten right-unilateral treatments. He agreed to a trial of maintenance ECT in addition to treatment with medication and cognitive behavioral therapy. Maintenance ECT was administered once a week for the first month and then gradually tapered and stopped six months after he was discharged from the hospital. He tolerated maintenance ECT fairly well but did experience difficulties with recalling certain items related to his job. These memory problems gradually improved about three months after ECT was discontinued. Three years later, he is doing well while continuing with medications and occasional booster sessions of cognitive behavioral therapy.

Case 2   A severely catatonic, 42-year-old woman was admitted to a state psychiatric facility and given a diagnosis of schizophrenia. In her catatonic state, she refused to eat or drink, stood in a mute, statuelike position for hours at a time while staring at the wall, and occasionally ran several steps before halting and resuming her statuelike posture. A week later, she was involuntarily transferred to an academic hospital's psychiatry service because she was becoming dangerously dehydrated, resulting in changes in her heart rate and blood chemistry. The transfer was approved by a judge during an involuntary commitment hearing.

At the academic hospital, the patient was given fluids and nourishment through a nasogastric tube inserted through her nose and into her stomach. She was also given antipsychotic medications via the tube. Although her weight stabilized and she no longer was dehydrated due to the tube feedings, the patient showed only minimal response to the medications and she remained mute, refusing to eat or drink. Because of the severity of her symptoms and her failure to improve with antipsychotic medication, the treating psychiatrist requested a court hearing to consider involuntary ECT. The patient and her lawyer were present at the hearing. The judge, after considering the evidence and trying unsuccessfully to interview the woman, approved a course of up to 12 treatments. Following the second treatment, the patient started whispering that she was being monitored by the FBI and that she therefore needed to talk softly. After the third treatment, she started to eat and drink. The nasogastric tube was removed. After the fourth treatment, she was able to describe an elaborate delusional system involving the belief that she was being monitored and controlled by outside forces. She indicated that the walls of the hospital prevented the "control beams" from reaching her. After the sixth treatment, she was able to participate in discussions with the treatment team and acknowledged the possibility that some of her thoughts might be the result of her mind playing tricks on her. In addition, she was able to tell them about her past psychiatric history; she reported that similar symptoms had occurred periodically since she was 20 years old. She also indicated that, at times, she had done well on a specific antipsychotic medication. The psychiatrist started the patient on this medication and discontinued ECT after the ninth treatment. The patient developed enough insight into her illness that she agreed to sign into the hospital as a voluntary patient. After two more weeks of medications, she was well enough to be discharged from the hospital. Discharge planning included close follow-up with the help of a case manager.

These two cases represent somewhat dramatic but realistic examples of the types of patients treated with ECT and highlight several points. First, severe psychiatric disorders can be medical emergencies requiring rapid intervention. Suicide and risks from starvation and dehydration are very real problems faced by psychiatrists who treat seriously ill patients. Second, for severe mood and psychotic disorders, ECT is one of the most dramatic treatments used in psychiatry and can be lifesaving. ECT can also help patients who have failed to respond to other treatments or who are too ill medically or psychiatrically to wait several weeks for medications to become effective. ECT is the most rapidly acting psychiatric treatment available, and patients often exhibit benefits after only a few treatments. Third, ECT is usually administered with voluntary informed patient consent, and patients who have previously benefited from ECT often opt for it as a preferred mode of treatment if they become ill again. In some severe cases, however, ECT can be administered involuntarily following appropriate legal review. These types of cases almost always involve psychiatric symptoms that impose significant risk to the patient or to others in contact with the patient. Fourth, ECT does not cure any psychiatric disorder, and appropriate maintenance treatment with psychiatric follow-up, medications, and psychotherapy is critical following a successful course of treatment. In some cases, ECT itself can be used as a maintenance treatment. Finally, ECT is associated with side effects, including memory loss and confusion. After a course of treatment is discontinued, this cognitive impairment typically improves with time, although some patients may note more persistent defects in some areas of recall.

Vagus Nerve Stimulation

Since the late 1990s, there has been an explosion of interest in developing new brain stimulation methods for use in psychiatry. One of these new methods, vagus nerve stimulation (VNS), was originally used to treat epilepsy and has been shown to have anticonvulsant effects, much like ECT. It is estimated that more than 30,000 patients have been treated with VNS for epilepsy. The vagus nerve is connected to areas in the brain that are important for regulating seizures and mood. To administer VNS, an electrical pacemaker is implanted in a patient's chest during a surgical procedure and connected to the vagus nerve. When this nerve is stimulated repeatedly with certain patterns of electrical activity, it has some beneficial effects on depression. Indeed, clinical trials have shown modest benefit in refractory (nonresponsive) depression, and the method has since been approved for this purpose by the US Food and Drug Administration (USFDA).

An intriguing aspect of VNS (but one that requires a lot more study) is that patients who respond to this treatment usually take a while to respond (maybe 3–6 months or longer), but once they improve, the benefits may last for several years with continued stimulation. In early trials, only a small percentage of patients responded to VNS initially; this percentage increased over several months of treatment, and those who did well tended to maintain the benefits for up to two years. Anecdotal evidence suggests that the benefits may persist even longer. If this holds true in future well-designed clinical trials, it could make VNS very important for treating chronic depressions and may point to ways to overcome the high relapse rate in these patients.

In general, VNS is tolerated well by patients. Some of the most bothersome side effects involve infections near the site where the pacemaker is implanted and changes in voice quality (hoarseness) when the pacemaker is on. A potential drawback with VNS is that adjustments in stimulus may be required over time. Furthermore, pacemaker batteries eventually run down and require replacement, although this can be accomplished by a fairly simple surgical procedure.

Other Brain Stimulation Methods

Two other forms of brain stimulation are currently under development as potential treatments in psychiatry: repetitive transcranial magnetic stimulation (rTMS) and deep brain stimulation (DBS). Work is further along with rTMS, and early results are promising but far from conclusive. With rTMS, an electromagnet is placed on the patient's head and used to generate electrical currents that penetrate the skull into the outer layers of the brain. This stimulation can either excite or inhibit brain activity, depending on the frequency with which the magnetic pulses are administered. Importantly, and unlike ECT, rTMS does not require general anesthesia and does not involve the induction of a seizure. This makes it possible for rTMS to be administered in an office setting that is equipped to handle any unexpected side effects. Like ECT, rTMS is administered as a course of multiple treatments, usually five days a week over several weeks. Courses of at least 15 to 20 rTMS sessions are commonly used. Each treatment session lasts about 30 to 60 minutes. In general, there are fewer side effects with rTMS than with ECT, and rTMS does not require a large medical team to administer it. Nor does rTMS appear to cause memory problems or other lasting cognitive impairment, and this could prove to be a major advantage over ECT. It remains unclear, however, whether rTMS has the kind of impact on severe and refractory depression that ECT does. Thus, its place as a therapeutic modality in psychiatry remains undefined. Despite these limitations, a device for administering rTMS to refractory-depressed patients was approved by the USFDA in late 2008.

DBS is the latest addition to the brain stimulation methods. The use of DBS in psychiatry has developed, in part, as a result of the success of electrical stimulation in improving motor symptoms in Parkinson's disease, for which DBS has become an accepted form of treatment. As mentioned in Chapter 6, Helen Mayberg and colleagues drew on neuroimaging investigations of the brain circuits involved in depression to initiate a bold study in which they targeted DBS to a specific region of prefrontal cortex that has abnormal activity in depressed patients. In a small number of patients with very refractory depression, they saw encouraging results with sustained benefits in several of these patients as long as electrical stimulation was maintained. DBS represents the most invasive of the brain stimulation methods and requires a neurosurgical procedure to implant electrodes in the patient's brain. There are clearly many ethical and clinical concerns about this form of treatment, but based on early results, the work is moving ahead. The use of DBS in depression potentially represents a new era for psychiatry: This is the first time that results from neuroimaging studies have paved the way to a new treatment and thus serves as an early proof of concept for the importance of neuroimaging in developing new therapies. Clinical studies of DBS for treating severe obsessive-compulsive disorder (OCD) are also in progress and have shown initial encouraging results. Based on early results, the USFDA approved an implantable DBS device for use in severe OCD in early 2009.

There are other forms of brain stimulation therapy currently under development. These include magnetic seizure therapy (MST) and focal electrically administered seizure therapy (FEAST). These involve attempts to use magnetic (MST) or electrical pulses (FEAST) to induce seizure activity in focal (localized) regions of the neocortex. These focal seizures secondarily generalize to the whole brain and thus are expected to have effects similar to those of ECT. The hope is that MST and/or FEAST will cause fewer side effects than ECT because of the more restricted areas of the brain stimulated. At this time, neither MST nor FEAST is approved for clinical use.

Psychosurgery

In the context of our discussion of DBS, we should also mention the use of other neurosurgical interventions in psychiatry (popularly referred to by the misnomer *lobotomies*). In these interventions, neurosurgeons employ sophisticated and precise methods to target specific regions of the prefrontal cortex, somewhat akin to the approach used in DBS. The surgical interventions alter the activity and connections of the targeted brain regions. Patients considered for psychosurgery usually have extremely refractory and debilitating major depression or OCD. Even so, psychosurgery represents the most invasive and drastic of all treatments in psychiatry, and it is used very rarely these days. Only a few centers actually do these procedures, and most modern psychiatrists have not had contact with patients who have undergone this intervention. Unfortunately, psychosurgery was used more frequently, and often inappropriately, before the psychopharmacology era. This remains one of the dark times in the history of psychiatry. Today, surgical interventions are only undertaken with extreme caution and after careful systematic review by psychiatrists and neurosurgeons working closely with patients and their families.

Take-Home Messages

- ECT can play a critical role in treating severe and refractory psychiatric disorders. Among the brain stimulation methods, ECT has by far the most data to support its use and the best track record. For hospitalized patients with severe depression, ECT is the "gold standard" against which other treatments must be compared. In some cases, ECT is truly a lifesaving intervention.

- Although ECT has marked beneficial effects and may be the only treatment that works for some patients, it is far from perfect and has significant side effects. The major issue for most patients is memory loss. As administered today in leading medical centers, however, ECT is a very safe procedure. ECT technique is geared toward increasing efficacy and diminishing risks, including the risks of cognitive impairment.

- The other brain stimulation methods—VNS, rTMS, and DBS in particular—are all in their infancy and require much more research before their place among psychiatric treatments is defined. We caution people to be skeptical about any mental health professionals who seem to be making claims about these treatments that sound too good to be true. In our opinion, VNS, rTMS, and DBS are experimental tools and are not ready for prime time . . . yet.

$\cdots$ eleven $\cdots$

How Can Patients and Families Help with Treatment?

The Importance of Educated Consumers

One of our goals in writing this book is to make psychiatry understandable to people who are not mental health professionals. The more patients and their families and friends know about psychiatric disorders and their treatments, including the roles of psychiatrists and other mental health professionals, the better it is for improving outcomes. Knowledge about the signs and symptoms of various disorders can go a long way toward the early recognition of imminent relapses. For example, a patient with bipolar mood disorder who begins to make repeated phone calls in the middle of the night is likely to be relapsing. Similarly, a person who is beginning to withdraw from interactions with friends and is giving up usual social activities could be exhibiting the early signs of major depression. Getting such individuals into treatment early is in everyone's best interest. Most disorders involving the nervous system do not improve, and often worsen, when left unchecked for long periods of time. This is true whether the disorder is epilepsy, Alzheimer's disease, or any of the psychiatric disorders. Left untreated, brain disorders tend to become more severe and more difficult to treat. While this is less clear for psychiatric disorders than for neurological disorders, we believe the principles hold true across specialties.

We also think it is important for people to understand what psychiatrists do and why they ask the questions they do. Psychiatrists are not mind readers or magicians, and they require help from patients and their families in order to provide effective care. Similarly, when patients understand why psychiatrists prescribe the treatments they do—medications, psychotherapies, and social interventions—it is a big help with overall management. The more patients know about these various interventions, the more they will know about what to expect from each one.

Psychiatric disorders are generally long-term problems. With some exceptions, patients are usually referred to psychiatrists when they have either developed severe symptoms or failed to respond to simple treatments. Thus, psychiatrists typically don't treat individuals who have only one bout of a disorder. Such individuals do exist, but they are not the norm in most psychiatric practices. As such, psychiatrists usually expect to be involved for the long haul in the care of their patients. It also bears repeating that there are *no cures* for psychiatric disorders. Syndromes and symptoms usually improve with treatment and can be put into complete remission with effective treatment. However, this does not mean that the underlying disorders are completely gone and will never recur. Often they do recur, and in some cases, treatment will be a life-long issue. Not understanding this point leads to a lot of patient dissatisfaction and a worsening of one's problems over time.

As stated in previous chapters, the causes of psychiatric disorders are not well understood. It is known, however, that single genes do not cause these illnesses. Thus, if someone in your family has schizophrenia or bipolar disorder, your risk and your children's risk are increased, but many other variables intervene, including many genetic and environmental factors. This circumstance makes it difficult to predict whether the disorder will occur in other family members. Psychiatrists may try to explain the causes of a disorder, often in an attempt to diminish the guilt and stigma that patients and families often feel about a given diagnosis, but these explanations generally are not statements of absolute scientific fact. In the final analysis, you can't control what genes you inherit or what environment you grow up in, but you can control what you know about psychiatric disorders and you can help in the management of the disorder that you or a family member or friend may have. Repeating a theme running throughout this book, the lack of knowledge about the mechanisms that cause disorders is not unique to psychiatry; it pervades all of medicine and neurology, particularly with regard to common disorders. But again, the good news is that treatments are available, and while not perfect, they can be highly effective.

Treatment Compliance

One of the most important things patients can do is to follow through with recommended treatments. Noncompliance with treatment kills clinical effectiveness and makes it difficult for any physician to determine a course of action if a patient's symptoms persist or worsen. Decisions about treatment are always collaborations between psychiatrists and patients. It is inappropriate for psychiatrists to dictate unilaterally one type of treatment for any given patient—one size does not fit all, and there are many paths to a successful outcome. This abundance of treatment options is one of the beauties of psychiatry and one of the reasons some physicians choose psychiatry as their area of specialty. It is equally inappropriate, however, for patients to decide to stop treatment on their own or to decide unilaterally that a treatment is not working. If patients have trouble with a given treatment choice, they must share their concerns with their psychiatrists in order to determine the most effective strategies. There are many problems with all current treatments in psychiatry, just as there are problems with treatments in all of medicine. Successful treatment is always a balance between the benefits of treatment and the risks of side effects or the risks of no treatment at all. Psychiatrists are accustomed to dealing with these issues and to working with their patients to correct problems and find better approaches. But they can't help if their patients don't follow through with a chosen approach. Thus, while being an educated, questioning consumer is essential to the treatment process, being a noncompliant one undermines the process and advances no one's interests, least of all the consumer's.

Compared with physicians in other branches of medicine, psychiatrists deal with some unique problems with regard to treatment compliance. Because psychiatric disorders are associated with problems in motivation, thinking, and judgment, psychiatrists often deal with patients who have little insight into the need for treatment, don't want treatment, or are suspicious of treatment. These are major obstacles for compliance. Here, educated and supportive families and friends can be critical, in effect helping with care during difficult periods. Blaming patients for compliance problems is not helpful, and support and guidance can go a long way toward helping patients to follow through with treatment. Because psychiatric disorders are long-term problems, it is also important that consumers understand that treatment should not be stopped once symptoms improve. The risk of relapse is extremely high if treatment of any of these disorders is terminated prematurely. Again, in some cases, life-long treatment will be necessary.

The Importance of Lifestyle: A Reprise

In Chapter 1, we discussed some of the leading causes of death in the United States, including several lifestyle variables, such as cigarette use, alcohol and drug use, sedentary activity, and obesity. Although some of these factors may reflect underlying psychiatric disorders, efforts to limit their presence can be extremely beneficial, improving not only a patient's general health but also the outcome of his or her psychiatric dysfunction. In these efforts, too, patients and their families play a critical role.

As discussed in a later chapter, one of the hopeful stories in psychiatry involves current research on neurogenesis, that is, on the birth of new nerve cells in the adult brain. Several factors help produce and sustain new nerve cells in adults, including a number of effective psychiatric treatments, such as certain medications (antidepressants in particular), and several environmental variables, such as exercise, diet, and learning. In Chapters 8 and 9, we touched on how patients can influence a few of these environmental variables in their own lives, and these points warrant brief reiteration here. The first point is related to exercise. One of the problems for many patients with psychiatric disorders is that they decrease or cease their normal activities, such as going to work, attending school, and pursuing hobbies, when they get ill. This behavior largely results from the underlying psychiatric disorder and certainly does not help its outcome. In fact, giving up activities and becoming sedentary not only don't help outcome, they likely make it worse. Thus, when therapists use cognitive behavioral therapy (CBT) with patients, the first emphasis is usually on the "B" word, *behavior*. That is, patients are encouraged to be as active as possible and are assigned homework that increases their activity level. This can be done in small steps at first, as in just getting out of bed in the morning, for example. Gradually, patients are expected to engage in increasing amounts of activity and self-care. This increased activity can have a positive impact on mood.

Ideally, getting patients to engage in forms of exercise also is important, as long as the type of exercise is within the realm of what the patient's underlying medical status will permit. Increased exercise could be as simple as walking about the house or around the block. To the extent that patients can increase their activity level, they can help their psychiatric symptoms. Some evidence suggests that exercise programs have positive effects on major depression, but there is no reason that this effect should be limited to depression. Simply put, there is little evidence that inactivity improves any chronic medical or psychiatric disorder. Anyone who has had a significant illness or injury understands this very well; even with chronic illnesses, patients are usually advised to avoid staying in bed and to become active as soon as possible and to the extent possible. Psychiatric disorders are no exception.

Diet is also an important consideration. Our diets, particularly those reliant upon fast foods, are notoriously bad for health. In turn, weight gain has adverse effects on activity and the overall outcome of any medical disorder. Patients can work with their psychiatrists and internists to improve their diets, which is likely to have beneficial effects overall. In effect, some degree of caloric restriction is likely to be good for you, and improving the quality of what you eat is likely to help a host of medical conditions.

Cigarette, alcohol, and illicit drug use can also be big problems for psychiatric patients. In some cases, substance abuse goes hand in hand with such psychiatric disorders as depression, schizophrenia, and bipolar disorder. There is no evidence that use of these agents helps the overall health of a person with any psychiatric disorder, and in fact, evidence is strong to the contrary. Moreover, substance abuse is one of the major contributors to bad outcomes in psychiatric disorders, leading to poor response to treatment, chronic symptoms, and noncompliance with treatment. Kicking these habits can be very difficult, particularly nicotine dependence. But again, if patients work with their psychiatrists to eliminate the use of these substances, overall benefits to health and mental state are likely to accrue.

Sleep, or more accurately sleep hygiene, is another lifestyle factor that can influence psychiatric symptoms. Many psychiatric disorders are associated with sleep disturbances, ranging from the difficulties in falling or staying asleep that occur in major depression to the diminished need for sleep that occurs in mania. Drug and alcohol abuse also are often accompanied by disrupted sleep. In the case of mood disorders, it is sometimes unclear whether the sleep problem is simply a symptom of the disorder or an attempt by the body to heal itself. There is some evidence that some forms of sleep deprivation can have short-term beneficial effects in major depression, whereas sleep deprivation can trigger manic episodes in patients with bipolar disorder.

Sleep problems can also affect emotion control and can exacerbate symptoms in individuals with psychiatric disorders. Psychiatric disorders often reflect dysregulation of emotional processing systems in the brain. These systems are important for determining our ability to assess situations rapidly and to make rapid adjustments that enhance our survival. For example, fear can be processed rapidly and nonconsciously to allow us to avoid danger. But these systems are capable of supercharging our brains and can in effect take over our ability to function appropriately. Our ability to control our emotions can require what is called "top-down processing" by cognitive scientists. This means that our higher cognitive centers in the prefrontal cortex sometimes must work consciously to keep emotions under wraps in inappropriate situations. This cognitive control takes mental effort, but when we are tired or physically drained, our emotions can run amok. Those who are fans of international soccer may have witnessed a glaring example of this in the 2006 World Cup final, when the French star Zinedane Zidane head-butted an opponent as time was winding down in the game. Physical fatigue may well have played a major role in this breakdown of emotional control for even a highly trained and highly fit world-class professional athlete. As all of us become physically and mentally tired, we become more "emotional." For these reasons, efforts aimed at improving sleep can be important in helping us to control our emotions. Simply stated, better sleep leads to improved energy and stronger emotional resolve.

Lifestyles in the United States contribute a lot to disrupting not only our diet and activity level but also our sleep-wake cycles. Examples range from variable shift work in some jobs to very bad sleep habits in general. It is common for psychiatrists and internists to prescribe sleep medications to help with these problems, but these medications are really short-term solutions and can create as many problems as they solve in the longer term. Alternatively, it is possible for patients to improve their sleep by working on their sleep hygiene. This includes setting regular times for sleeping and waking, avoiding daytime naps, minimizing caffeine use, removing televisions and food from bedrooms, and making sure the bedroom is a comfortable and calm setting. To the extent that patients take responsibility for their sleep habits and environment, they do themselves a favor that will probably result in significant benefit.

Psychotherapy and Learning

Learning is good for your brain. It enhances your nervous system by creating new connections among neurons and by strengthening existing connections. Learning also is associated with the growth of new neurons in the brain. In this sense, your brain can get "bigger" with learning. A great example of this comes from a study of taxi drivers in London and highlights the key role that the hippocampus plays in the ability to learn new information (e.g., spatial relationships). These taxi drivers rely on detailed mental maps in order to navigate London's highly complex road system. It turns out that they appear to have larger hippocampi compared to the rest of us; this likely reflects their mastery of this form of complex spatial learning. Extrapolating from this study, we believe that treatments such as psychotherapy are all about learning. In psychotherapy, patients are taught to think about their symptoms and problems and are encouraged to find solutions. Thus, voluntary participation in various forms of psychotherapy is a good way for patients to help themselves, particularly when they try to incorporate into their daily lives what they learn in therapy.

It is less clear whether other forms of learning are beneficial in psychiatric disorders. However, we would argue that learning in general is a good thing for the brain. Thus, taking courses, including self-help courses, can be advantageous. It is also possible that doing puzzles and mental games in adulthood can help delay age-related cognitive changes. Higher educational achievement earlier in life is associated with a protective effect against Alzheimer's disease later in life. We do not believe that it is a great extrapolation to extend these findings to other psychiatric disorders where defects in cognition are common. With regard to our brains, the old adage seems true—"use it or lose it." What has also become clear in geriatric medicine is that a lifestyle of passive TV watching and Internet surfing is not good for the brain. Furthermore, retirement from one's job, if not accompanied by maintenance of social activities, hobbies, and interests, can be extremely bad for humans. Openness to lifelong learning and cognitive activity can be good for all of us.

Social Networks

Humans are inherently social animals. We live in social environments, and our well being is often tied to the strength of our connectedness to others. Being isolated from society or losing our social network is bad for our overall function and mental health. A sad feature of many psychiatric disorders is that they often disrupt social ties and diminish a person's desire to remain in contact with others. Clear examples include the withdrawn nature of many patients with schizophrenia, the withdrawal from friends and family that can accompany depression, and even the fear of being around people or places that is associated with social phobia or agoraphobia. Another example is the tendency among alcoholics to drink alone.

In none of these cases is social withdrawal good for the individual, and in fact, loss of social contact can be a factor contributing to suicide risk. The French behavioral scientist Émile Durkheim studied social contributors to suicide and believed that for some individuals suicide reflected a breakdown in their ability to function within their culture. Durkheim referred to this as "anomic suicide." Thus, in treating some patients, efforts aimed at improving social function and social contact can be very important. This contact can be crucial for both ensuring follow-up for care and providing a type of interpersonal safety net for the individual. One example is the use of groups like Alcoholics Anonymous in treating alcoholics. In other cases, group therapy, clubhouse rehabilitation settings, and even community-based case workers can be important for providing patients with positive forms of social connectedness. Churches and social organizations can also provide meaningful social connection. To the extent that patients and their families and friends recognize the importance of human contact and work to maintain social contacts, they can help to avoid the isolation that often accompanies severe psychiatric disorders. As is true for all the lifestyle factors we have discussed, social contact will not cure psychiatric dysfunction, but it can go a long way toward diminishing some complications of the illnesses and in helping the healing process. This is another variable that can be possibly controlled and enhanced by patients and their social network.

Take-Home Messages

- By becoming educated consumers, patients, families, and friends can greatly assist in the diagnosis, treatment, and outcome of psychiatric disorders. Psychiatrists can facilitate the education process by teaching about the signs, symptoms, and treatment of psychiatric disorders. In some cases, patients will need the help of their families and friends when illness disrupts insight and judgment.

- Poor treatment compliance and failure to persist with follow-up care are major factors contributing to poor outcomes for patients with psychiatric disorders. To the extent possible, patients should take responsibility for continued follow-up care and compliance. Help with follow-up care from the patient's social network can be important as well.

- Patients can greatly help the management of their psychiatric disorders by improving their lifestyle in several specific ways, including better diet, increased exercise, and better sleep habits. Limiting cigarette use and alcohol and illicit drug intake also is very important. Drug and alcohol abuse are strong predictors of poor outcome in all psychiatric disorders.

- Efforts to maintain beneficial social networks can be important in providing support and help for patients with psychiatric disorders. At times, this will be difficult for family and friends because certain psychiatric disorders, by their very nature, disrupt patients' desire for human contact. Nonetheless, humans typically do not do well when socially isolated. Thus, efforts to maintain and enhance social contacts and activities are in everyone's best interest.

··· *twelve* ···

Consumers Beware

A recurring theme in this book has been that psychiatric disorders involve abnormal brain function and are serious medical problems. Complications from these disorders can be devastating for individuals, families, and society, and can include suicide, violence, physical abuse, premature death from a variety of causes, job loss, and discord in relationships. Thus, we believe that psychiatric disorders merit the highest level of attention from the highest-quality providers in our health care delivery system.

Like all of medicine, psychiatry boasts a large number of outstanding clinicians who use evidence-based approaches to diagnose and treat their patients. These clinicians provide extremely high levels of care to patients and their families. However, as in all of medicine, some practices in psychiatry and the mental health care delivery system are less evidenced based than others and may be questionable in their benefit or utility for patients. It can be extremely difficult for patients and their families to know the difference, however, and so in this chapter, we will discuss some practices that we believe should raise red flags in the minds of consumers.

Practitioners Vary Widely in Their Training and Expertise

Earlier we described the training of psychiatrists, which includes medical school, residency, and in some cases, post-residency fellowships. In order to practice medicine, all psychiatrists must obtain medical licenses from their state medical boards. These licenses reflect the qualifications of the physician to practice medicine in general. They indicate that the physician has successfully completed medical school, has had at least some post-medical school training, and has passed at least some general qualifying examinations, like the examinations from the National Board of Medical Examiners. However, state medical licenses do not indicate whether a physician has successfully completed a residency program in psychiatry. As noted previously, some psychiatrists are certified by the American Board of Psychiatry and Neurology (ABPN). This "board certification" indicates that a psychiatrist has completed medical school and psychiatry residency training in an approved program and has passed a qualifying examination in psychiatry administered by the ABPN. For most psychiatrists, maintenance of medical license and board certification requires participation in ongoing continuing medical education. Thus, one marker of a psychiatrist's level of training and ongoing education is ABPN certification. Some psychiatrists who train in such subspecialty areas as child and adolescent psychiatry, geriatric psychiatry, forensic psychiatry, and addiction psychiatry maintain subspecialty board certification in those areas as well, although this is not required for general psychiatric practice.

It is important to emphasize that psychiatrists are only one segment of the mental health delivery system. A large number of practitioners are psychologists (who have master's or doctoral, i.e., PhD or equivalent, degrees), social workers (who often have master's or doctoral degrees), and counselors. The training of these other mental health professionals can vary widely, particularly in the general field of "counseling." Some form of state licensure is required to practice, but the degree of training, expertise, and post-training monitoring can be quite different from place to place. In some locales, being called a "psychologist" may have little to do with the actual training and experience of the individual. A recent analysis by Thomas Insel, Director of the National Institute of Mental Health, highlights this concern and indicates that at least half of the training programs for social workers and psychologists do not emphasize evidence-based approaches to clinical care. Evidenced-based approaches refer to those interventions that have the highest degree of empirical support in well-designed clinical trials.

Based on these considerations, understanding the credentials of any and all mental health professionals is a good place for patients and families to start when choosing a mental health care provider. Local medical and other boards can be sources of information. Whether a professional holds privileges in a local hospital system is also a marker of scrutiny by the hospital's credentialing committee. Among mental health professionals, only psychiatrists are able to prescribe medications and electroconvulsive therapy independently. Advanced practice nurses and physician's assistants are allowed to prescribe medications, but only under the supervision of a physician. Patients should be extremely cautious about nonphysician providers who claim to have the expertise to prescribe medications independently.

The Vagaries of Psychiatric Diagnoses

Throughout this book, we have pointed out a number of areas where psychiatry is making great progress, including advances in psychiatric diagnosis dating back to 1980, when the third edition of the *Diagnostic and Statistical Manual of Mental Disorders* (DSM-III) was published. But we have also pointed out that not all psychiatric diagnoses are equal in terms of the amount of information they convey to other health professionals and that validation of the diagnoses at the level of uncovering the underlying mechanisms lags behind other fields of medicine. Many of the major diagnoses in psychiatry have been reasonably well validated based on a set of criteria initially proposed by Eli Robins and Sam Guze at Washington University in the early 1970s. Disorders that adhere to these validation criteria have a clear clinical description, are differentiated from other psychiatric and medical conditions, have a pattern of symptoms that can be recognized over the long-term course of the disorder, and tend to run in families.

Examples of well-validated psychiatric diagnoses include major depression, bipolar (type I) disorder, schizophrenia, panic disorder, obsessive-compulsive disorder, alcoholism, somatization disorder (Briquet's syndrome), and antisocial personality disorder, among others. Some very popular diagnoses are much less well validated, including multiple personality disorder (dissociative identity disorder), borderline personality disorder, seasonal mood disorder, premenstrual syndrome, conversion disorder, and some forms of posttraumatic stress disorder (PTSD), among others. This is not to say that these are not real disorders, but rather that they are less well studied and understood and that the predictive validity of these diagnoses is less certain. In these cases, it is often not clear that the disorder follows a predictable course and that the current symptoms are not better explained by another, better validated psychiatric diagnosis or even medical disorder. This is a complicated topic, but it is one that can lead to useful discussions among patients, families, and their mental health treatment team when questions about diagnosis, treatment, and course of illness arise.

That many of the major (and most common) psychiatric disorders are well validated does not mean that scientists yet understand the underlying biological mechanisms of these disorders. They don't, at least not yet. Nor are there *any* laboratory tests or neuroimaging studies that are diagnostic of *any* psychiatric disorder (at least as of 2009). Laboratory tests and imaging studies can be very useful for determining the presence of medical or neurological disorders that contribute to, or in some cases cause, a patient's symptoms. But these tests, no matter how scientific they may sound, cannot prove the existence of any specific psychiatric disorder. Thus, consumers should be wary of psychiatrists or other mental health providers who claim that they can use sophisticated-sounding lab studies to determine whether the patient has a specific disorder. Although this claim can sound very scientific, it is often nonsense.

One clear example of this was the use of "brain electrical activity monitoring" (BEAM) by some psychiatrists in the past. BEAM generates very pretty pictures of brain activity that generally have nothing to do with the psychiatric disorder being treated. Other brain imaging studies can be presented in an array of amazing computer-generated colors, called "pseudocoloring," in order to highlight findings of interest. Although the results of these imaging studies look impressive, they may not convey much useful information. Some scientists have used a wonderful phrase to express their dismay about some of the brain imaging studies done in psychiatry, referring to them as "pseudo-color phrenology." Phrenology is the now-discredited "science" of the past that diagnosed personality and psychiatric problems by analyzing bumps on a patient's skull. This discussion is not meant to demean the future prospects for neuroimaging in psychiatry or the importance of brain imaging in determining the presence of certain neurological disorders, such as brain tumors or strokes. The hope is that imaging studies and genetic profiles will be useful in the future for diagnosing psychiatric disorders, but the field isn't there yet.

Some practitioners also use a variety of psychological tests to make diagnoses and decide on treatment approaches. Presently, it is unclear whether these instruments really provide much additional diagnostic information over that provided by a thorough clinical examination. Certain psychological tests, particularly neuropsychological tests such as the Halstead-Reitan Battery or the Wechsler Intelligence or Memory Tests, can be very helpful in understanding deficits in a patient's cognitive and intellectual function and in determining whether such deficits are changing over time. These tests survey a range of intellectual functions, including verbal skills, nonverbal aspects of memory, and the ability to detect spatial relationships. Similarly, certain personality instruments such as the Minnesota Multiphasic Personality Inventory (MMPI)—a test that has been well validated in a large number of studies—can be helpful in understanding the range of symptoms and personality traits that patients display. Other tests, including some that are popular in certain segments of the mental health community, such as the Rorschach Test (interpreting inkblots) and the Thematic Apperception Test (TAT; describing a story when presented with a picture), are of dubious use. These two instruments are called "projective tests," which means that individuals project their own thinking and feelings into what they report when presented with a fairly nonspecific stimulus. The problem with these tests lies in how to interpret reliably and validly the information patients describe during testing. The use of anatomically correct dolls to detect sexual abuse is another example of a test that has little proven validity either as a diagnostic instrument or as an instrument to detect sexual abuse. Problems with these last three tests have been highlighted cogently by Lilienfeld and colleagues in their book, *Science and Pseudoscience in Clinical Psychology*.

The problem for consumers is how to distinguish real science from nonsense. Frank and open discussions with their mental health providers is a good first step. Again, we emphasize the importance of the practitioner's prior training and openness to engage in such informed dialogue with patients and their families. Consumers should be wary of practitioners who suggest a lot of tests and are making money from the use of these instruments, either for conducting these tests or for interpreting their results. Financial conflicts of interest among practitioners can be a significant problem in all of medicine and mental health.

Snake Oil and Psychiatric Treatments

Psychiatric treatments can be very effective in controlling symptoms and putting syndromes into remission, and they can be lifesaving for many individuals. Nevertheless, these treatments aren't perfect, and they are not cures: They cannot eliminate the cause of the disorder and its associated abnormal physiology. Psychiatric disorders are "managed" and are generally long-term problems. They usually don't arise overnight, and they usually don't go away overnight. Treatment is often a long-term and sometimes life-long undertaking. Thus, consumers should beware of practitioners who claim that they can cure these complex disorders either with medications or with psychotherapies. It just doesn't happen. In days of yore, there were hucksters who went from town to town proclaiming amazing cures for a variety of common maladies. These individuals were in it for the money and often sold a variety of "treatments" that were derogatorily referred to as "snake oil." We have not evolved beyond the existence of such individuals, and today we still have an amazing number of snake oil salespersons, some of whom masquerade as mental health professionals. The point we want to make is this: Be careful about outrageous claims on the part of any "professional." If what they promise sounds too good to be true, it probably is. This includes a substantial part of the "self-help" industry that provides patients with a host of ways to cure everything from anxiety to psychosis. We would also suggest caution regarding providers who tout their way of treatment as the "only way." For example, some therapists and support groups advocate that their clients *never* take *any* psychiatric medications. Such statements reflect a serious misunderstanding of the nature and treatment of psychiatric illnesses. Patients and families are strongly advised to avoid such practitioners.

The "snake oil" problem can rear its head in another way in medicine and psychiatry. Some practitioners work for the pharmaceutical industry and are paid significant sums of money to consult with, speak for, and/or conduct clinical studies on behalf of drug companies. In most cases, this relationship is healthy and important both for developing new medications and for determining new directions in treatment. In some cases, however, the financial relationships can create major conflicts of interest for treating physicians. This has become a significant problem for some practitioners and has led to a number of high-profile cases in the news. In many academic medical centers, concerns about conflicts of interest have led to the institution of formal policies monitoring the relationships that doctors have with industry and, in cases where there is significant potential for conflict, requiring physicians to notify their patients about these relationships. Thus, at most academic centers, there are at least some, albeit imperfect, reporting and monitoring. Generally, however, this is not the case in private practice settings. Here patients may be prescribed treatments or even be enrolled in industry-supported clinical drug trials without knowing that their doctors are involved financially with the companies that make the medications these doctors are recommending and that sponsor the studies they are conducting. Most patients feel awkward about asking their doctors about industry relationships, so it seems most appropriate that physicians let their patients know when they have potential conflicts. All humans are subject to bias, and physicians are no exception. Patients deserve to know about these potential biases and their possible influence on the care their doctors provide. Patients should expect an open discussion about these issues with their physicians.

Faddism, Bad Logic, and Psychiatry

The fact that little is understood presently about why psychiatric disorders occur has not stopped some practitioners (and even patients and the general public) from making strong statements about what causes these disorders. The human brain is very good at coincidence detection; this is how we learn and remember. Things that happen close together in time are wired together by our brains. Humans are also notoriously adept at turning that coincidence into cause; think about various superstitions as examples.

But coincidence does not mean cause. It just means that things occur together. Demonstrating causality requires carefully controlled experiments in which specific variables are manipulated one at a time while the other variables are held constant.

In psychiatry, stress and life events are great examples of how coincidence and cause can be confused. There is no doubt that bad things happen to people and can sometimes precipitate psychiatric distress. The issue of cause is complicated, however, because having a psychiatric disorder is also stressful and can result in bad life events. This creates a complicated "chicken-and-egg" problem where it is often difficult to figure out what came first: the disorder or the adverse events. Thus, one has to be careful about making bold statements about "cause" and "effect" and about jumping to premature conclusions. Importantly, this can be as much of a problem for mental health professionals and physicians as it is for patients because clinicians are not taught to be experimental scientists and the logic in the clinical and experimental science worlds is not the same. Clinicians in all fields are taught to think about diagnosis and patient care; they are not taught to think about cause and effect in a rigorous, scientific way.

The "recovered memories" story of the last few decades is a major example where seeking "causes" for psychiatric dysfunction led people astray. The term *recovered memories* refers to events, often traumatic, that patients remember only after substantial prodding from their therapists or under hypnosis. In many of these cases, it was later determined that the "recovered memories" reflected events that never actually happened. In the meantime, patients and their therapists became convinced that the events were real, and this led to major discord among families and friends who tried to defend themselves against accusations that they knew were false.

How can people "remember" things that never happened? To answer this, it is important to understand how human memory works. Our brains are neither computers nor cameras. What people remember is a complex mixture of actual events and their own interpretation about the past and present. Individuals recall their own memories as "truth," but one person's version of the "truth" may not agree with the observations of an impartial outside observer. This problem is discussed in great detail by psychologist Daniel Schacter in his wonderful book, *The Seven Sins of Memory*. Schacter highlights multiple ways that our memories fool us. Sometimes, a person simply forgets things or remembers things the wrong way because of coincidences.

Furthermore, when forming memories, people are subject to a host of their own biases and misattributions that flavor what actually happened. The human brain is highly suggestible and tends to fill in the blanks to make up for missing information. Thus, individuals can "remember" many things that may or may not be real and can convince themselves that things did indeed happen when they really didn't. This has been found to be true with eyewitness testimony in legal cases. The sad part of the "recovered memory" story as it relates to psychiatry is not that patients were induced to have false memories, but that the so-called professional therapists failed to realize what they were doing and believed more in their own psychological ideology than in real science and logic. This resulted in a major embarrassment for the field. Fortunately, this fad appears to have faded, but patients should be wary that some other version of this pseudoscientific lunacy may rear its head in the future.

We would like to highlight one more area of concern. This one falls under the subtitle of "better living through chemistry" and involves the fallacy that psychiatric medications can actually control or cure *all* symptoms and conditions. The corollary to this belief is that "if a little is good, a lot is better." Our concern here is with the disturbing tendency of some psychiatrists to overprescribe psychiatric medications, particularly by using multiple medications for a single patient. We've mentioned this practice before, and it's called "polypharmacy." In some cases, the use of multiple medications from different drug categories that have different mechanisms makes a lot of sense. In these cases, "rational" polypharmacy can be highly effective and relieve symptoms not otherwise well managed. But in other cases, physicians prescribe medications in a way that is hard to justify, including using multiple drugs of the same type in the same patient, for example, using Valium (diazepam) together with Xanax (alprazolam) for anxiety or prescribing several antidepressants of a similar class to treat depression. Importantly, there is *no* treatment in all of medicine that has *no* side effects. (This actually includes placebos or "sugar pills.") The more medications a patient takes, the higher the probability that the patient will experience at least one major side effect from at least one of the medications. Furthermore, the evidence that this "irrational" polypharmacy enhances clinical response is sketchy at best and nonexistent in most cases.

Again, treatment decisions regarding any medical disorder should reflect close collaboration between the patient and the doctor. Consumers must beware of practitioners who spend little time with them and who are quick to reach for their prescription pad. A thorough discussion about the benefits and risks of all treatments should be part of every doctor–patient relationship. Patients can also help in the decision-making process by understanding that more is not necessarily better when it comes to the number and doses of medications. Unrealistic expectations and demands on the part of patients can contribute to inappropriate polypharmacy, and ultimately, it is the patient who pays the price . . . in more ways than one. Similarly, patients should follow through with treatment recommendations as prescribed by their doctors and be truthful with their doctors when they don't. Odd and complex medication regimens in all of medicine sometimes reflect a physician's efforts to deal with unrecognized poor treatment compliance on the part of the patient.

Take-Home Messages

- Most psychiatric practitioners and therapists do great jobs caring for their patients and employ state-of-the-art evidence-based treatments. Not all practitioners are the same, however, and there can be tremendous variability in quality, expertise, education, and experience.

- There is some inherent uncertainty in psychiatric diagnoses, reflecting both the lack of knowledge regarding underlying mechanisms and the overlap among disorders. Diagnoses in psychiatry are based on careful and repeated evaluations of the patient. Laboratory tests may play a role in helping to diagnose complicating medical or neurological disorders, but at this time, laboratory tests by themselves do not diagnose psychiatric disorders.

- There have been fads in the mental health field that have caused significant problems. Again, patients must become educated consumers, and patient education should be a priority for all mental health professionals. If the explanations given by a provider seem mystical or unrealistic, patients should be cautious and get another opinion.

- Choices about treatment should always be collaborations between patients and their mental health providers. No one approach or therapy fits all patients, and a dialogue with the provider can help patients and their families make informed decisions.

··· *thirteen* ···

Case Examples

The purpose of this chapter is to present several case examples in order to illustrate various principles that we discussed in earlier chapters. The individuals discussed in this chapter are not actual patients. Rather, we have created realistic and common scenarios drawn from our experience.

Case 1. Is This 20-Year-Old Student Having a Heart Attack?

A healthy 20-year-old college junior was doing well in all aspects of her life. School, although busy and stressful, was exciting. She was an A student. She had friends, a boyfriend, and a loving and supportive family. She was healthy other than being mildly inconvenienced by various food intolerances and mild irritable bowel disorder. Her weight was normal. She didn't exercise as much as she knew she should.

She was playing board games with friends on a Saturday night when suddenly she felt her heart skipping beats. She developed chest discomfort. She began to sweat and became afraid that she was having a heart attack. She started to breathe rapidly and felt numbness and tingling in her arms and legs. Her friends immediately called the school nurse who instructed them to call 911. She was brought to a local emergency room (ER). By the time she arrived, the symptoms had subsided. The ER doctor ordered an electrocardiogram (EKG) and some blood tests and did a careful physical exam. The doctor told the student that she was okay and that she should follow up with the doctors at her college's student health service.

A few days later, she had similar symptoms that lasted about 30 minutes. The doctor at the student health service referred her to a cardiologist who did another EKG, a stress test, and a careful physical exam. He said that her heart was fine and she should not worry.

Several months passed. The student was at one of her classes when she had another episode. She was afraid that she was dying, and she immediately left class and returned to her dorm. She felt better an hour later. Two days later, this happened in class again. She became afraid to go to class and increasingly stayed in her room. She started to become more withdrawn and to avoid her friends. She was afraid the doctors were wrong and that she had heart disease and was dying. She developed insomnia and didn't feel like eating. She couldn't concentrate on studying. She didn't go to class because she thought this provoked her "heart attacks."

Her friends became worried. They saw a dramatic change in her behavior. They decided to call her parents. Both parents drove to campus that night and took her home. The family doctor saw her the next day. He had known this young woman most of her life and knew how healthy she had been. He heard her story and thought that she might benefit from counseling. A counselor saw her a week later. The counselor was interested in working with the student but wanted a psychiatrist to evaluate her first. She saw a psychiatrist two weeks later. Meanwhile, she had had several "heart attacks" at home and continued to be sullen and worried.

The psychiatrist gathered all the information from the various doctors the student had seen and diagnosed panic disorder as well as a major depressive episode. The psychiatrist carefully explained the meaning of the diagnoses to the patient and her family. She told them that panic disorder is a common disorder and that it can be frightening. She further reassured them that the symptoms usually respond to medication and brief therapy. She explained that the medication she would prescribe, a selective serotonin reuptake inhibitor (SSRI), would take about four weeks to work. She also recommended that the patient set up appointments for cognitive behavioral therapy (CBT) with the counselor as well as a brief follow-up appointment with the psychiatrist in one week. The psychiatrist also suggested that the patient start a diary to document both the episodes and the patient's current activity at the time these episodes occurred.

Over the next eight weeks, the patient visited the psychiatrist three more times. The SSRI was increased in dosage, and the psychiatrist was calm and reassuring. The patient also had four sessions of CBT. After this eight-week period, the frequency of episodes diminished substantially, and the patient's depressive symptoms improved. Following the suggestion of the psychiatrist and the counselor, she and her mother sat in on some classes at a local college, and the student began to relax in the classroom setting.

She returned to school the next semester. Occasionally, she would have a single panic attack, but she now understood the nature of the disorder and didn't allow it to interfere with her activities. She continued to take the SSRI and did well.

This case illustrates the following principles:

- Emergency room doctors may not be able to tell patients exactly what is causing their symptoms. These doctors are trained to recognize serious illnesses, and they are very good at telling if a person's symptoms indicate a need for immediate attention. They may not have the expertise or the time to figure out nonemergency disorders.

- Primary care doctors are likely to think of physical ailments consistent with a person's symptoms prior to considering psychiatric disorders. They may or may not consider the role of psychiatric disorders in physical symptoms.

- Specialists, for example, cardiologists, evaluate what they know. They may or may not think of psychiatric disorders as causing symptoms, but they are very good at determining whether a set of signs and symptoms fits within their expertise.

- In this case, a doctor who knew the patient well realized that the disorder was psychiatric in nature. He referred her to a mental health counselor. Some primary care doctors refer to counselors; some utilize psychiatrists in order to establish a diagnosis.

- The counselor recognized that careful diagnosis was important and that treatment should be multidisciplinary. Hence the counselor asked for a psychiatric evaluation.

- The psychiatrist had enough history and information to make accurate diagnoses and initiate treatment. She utilized various treatment approaches, including medication, education, reassurance, being available, and referral back to the counselor for psychotherapy.

- Even though the student eventually did well, she lost a semester of school and suffered from undiagnosed symptoms for months. This was costly in many senses of the word.

Case 2. Is It Normal for a 58-Year-Old Man to Become a Couch Potato after a Heart Attack?

A 58-year-old man named Jim had a history of high blood pressure, high cho-lesterol, low thyroid function, and angina pectoris (chest pain on exertion). He had been a two-pack-a-day cigarette smoker for 40 years. Six months ago, he had a sudden onset of chest pain. He was immediately brought to the emer-gency room where a small myocardial infarction (heart attack) was diagnosed. One of Jim's coronary arteries was clogged, and the next day, the cardiologist placed a device called a stent into this artery in order to open it up and provide blood to the heart muscle. Jim was released from the hospital in four days and referred to a cardiac rehabilitation program. He took three drugs to keep his blood pressure under control, two drugs to lower his blood cholesterol, a thyroid medication, and aspirin, plus another blood thinner.

Jim stopped smoking and started attending the cardiac rehabilitation pro-gram. He worked with the cardiac rehabilitation staff to develop a program of exercise and good nutrition. But about six weeks after starting cardiac reha-bilitation, Jim stopped going. He began to smoke again. He became a couch potato and ate foods that he knew were bad for him (a lot of sweets and starches). He didn't have the energy or motivation to return to work, and he began to feel sorry for himself. His self-esteem plummeted. He was tired all the time. Although Jim had been passionate about sports and antique cars, he no longer was interested in either. He was not suicidal, but he felt that the future was bleak and that he no longer served any useful functions. His wife and adult children tried to get him involved in various activities, but he just couldn't push himself to participate in them.

A month later, he saw his cardiologist. The doctor thought that Jim's physi-cal recovery from the heart attack was excellent. However, he was concerned about Jim's mental health, and so the cardiologist's office staff made an appointment for Jim to see a consulting psychiatrist. Jim was uninterested in going. He did not think that he was "crazy" and did not want to see a "shrink." His wife, however, convinced him to keep the appointment.

Jim agreed to let his wife accompany him to his appointment with the psy-chiatrist and participate in the discussion. This psychiatrist had a lot of experi-ence working with patients who had had heart attacks, and he explained the common relationship between depression and heart disease. He told Jim and his wife that patients who had suffered heart attacks have a greater likelihood of future heart problems if they have an active depression. The psychiatrist kept the discussion at a very medical level. He recommended a trial of a par-ticular antidepressant that interacted very little with Jim's other medications and was known to be reasonably safe in patients with heart disease. He explained that the antidepressant took some time to work but that Jim should be feeling its effects gradually over the following several weeks. He further explained that the depression was probably responsible for Jim's lack of motivation, and so together they worked out a plan whereby Jim would return to cardiac rehabilitation a few days a week. The psychiatrist also recommended that Jim see him for frequent, brief follow-up visits, and Jim agreed. The psychiatrist also asked Jim to keep a diary of his daily activities.

Two weeks later, Jim reported that, although he had attended a few cardiac rehab sessions, he still wasn't very active. The psychiatrist reviewed Jim's activity diary with him and pointed out that Jim had started to be more interested in watching sports on TV and had exercised a bit more. At his appointment two weeks later, Jim reported being a bit more active, and he was able to smile and tell a humorous story about one of his grandkids. He was now participating routinely in cardiac rehabilitation. Two weeks after that, he reported that his gradual improvement continued, although he complained that he still tired easily. The psychiatrist explained that it takes many months to regain previous energy levels following even a mild heart attack. At this visit, the psychiatrist brought up the smoking issue, and Jim agreed to go to a smoking cessation group. Eventually, he agreed to try replacement therapy with nicotine patches, together with group therapy. Progress was gradual, but three months later, Jim had quit smoking cigarettes, was able to do cardiac exercises three times per week, and had returned part time to his engineering job. Six months later, Jim had returned to his normal activities, was eating well, and was not smoking. He was exercising routinely. A gradual decrease in the dose of antidepressant was initiated. After three more months, he continued to do well off of the antidepressant. He called the psychiatrist six months later to let him know that he was continuing to do well and that he was routinely exercising and couldn't stand cigarette smoke.

This case illustrates the following principles:

- Heart attacks are frequently time-linked to depression. In some cases, the depression precedes the heart attack; in other cases, the depression occurs following the heart attack. In both instances, depression can worsen the outcome of the cardiac disorder.

- Physical dysfunction can reinforce mental dysfunction and vice versa.

- Family encouragement to seek treatment for mental health can be critical.

- Psychiatrists have the flexibility to match the treatment approach to the patient. This patient was not excited about seeing a psychiatrist, so the psychiatrist decided to utilize a strictly medical approach.

- Timing is critical. If the psychiatrist had jumped on the smoking issue at the first visit, he might have alienated the patient. Waiting until the patient's depression had started to respond to treatment gave the patient time to become comfortable with the psychiatrist and to begin to feel better. He was then strong enough to work successfully on smoking cessation.

- The psychiatrist's approach involved integration of medications, cardiac rehab and exercise, support and education, and eventually a focus on the nicotine dependency.

Case 3. Do Multiple Physical Complaints Necessarily Signal the Presence of Severe Medical Illnesses?

Misty was sick a lot in high school. She had frequent physical complaints—stomach pain and episodes of nausea, severe menstrual pain, spells of weakness in her right arm and left leg, headaches, and pain involving her back and knees. She saw a variety of specialists, but no one could figure out the reasons for her problems. She had several exploratory surgeries, but no abnormalities were found. She missed enough school that it took her an extra year to finish high school.

Misty had rather a chaotic home situation and social life. Her father and brother were heavy drinkers. Her mother worked and tried to hold the family together. Misty had friends but often had fights with them. She had many boyfriends. These relationships often progressed rapidly from true love to vicious hate. She got bored easily. She would sometimes spread inaccurate gossip that caused her girlfriends to become angry with each other.

After high school, Misty got a job as a secretary. She tried to initiate an affair with her 40-year-old boss. When he indicated that he was happily married and was uninterested in a relationship with her, she became extremely angry and moody. She started to have repeated episodes in which she would cut her arm with a razor blade. She overdosed on Tylenol at work and then called her boss to tell him that he was the cause of her overdose. He called an ambulance, and Misty was evaluated at an emergency room. She had taken enough Tylenol that there was concern that she might have done harm to her liver. She was watched overnight, and by morning, she had recovered medically. She felt better after talking to the social worker and ER doctor, who referred her to a counselor for mental health follow-up.

She met with the counselor for several sessions. The counselor explored Misty's childhood with her and asked about childhood abuse. Initially, Misty denied that she was abused. However, the counselor returned frequently to this topic, and eventually Misty began to remember that she had been sexually abused by her uncle and her minister. She started to reveal graphic details about such abuse. Misty agreed to let the counselor talk with her family about this. After much investigation, it turned out that this abuse had never occurred.

Misty's life continued to be chaotic for several years. The counselor tried to help by exploring the meaning of Misty's behaviors, but Misty continued getting into trouble with jobs, friends, family, and boyfriends. She often cut her arms with a razor blade; she felt this relieved tension. She also continued to have many physical complaints, and she was angry that the doctors couldn't figure out what was wrong with her. Over the years, her doctors gave her a variety of diagnoses, including "fibromyalgia," and they treated her with a variety of pain medications, including Oxycontin.

When she was 32, Misty saw a surgeon for continued abdominal pain. The surgeon reviewed her entire history as well as the results from her earlier exploratory abdominal surgeries. He decided that she should see a psychiatrist prior to any more invasive procedures.

Misty saw a psychiatrist. She found the doctor extremely attractive and enjoyed her appointments. She tried to inquire into his personal life and figure out what he found attractive in women. The psychiatrist took a careful history of Misty's physical and behavioral symptoms. He diagnosed her as having somatization disorder and borderline personality disorder. The psychiatrist emphasized to Misty that her physical pains were very real but that they were caused by the way her mind interpreted pain. In other words, they didn't have a physical cause that could be found or cured. He explained that she could be harmed by having unnecessary procedures and by taking excessive amounts of medications. He suggested that he would help her to find an internist who could work with her to make sure that unnecessary medical procedures were not done. Also, as Misty got older, it was likely that other illnesses would develop, and thus, having a regular internist who could help Misty distinguish disorders caused by her brain's interpretation of pain from disorders caused by objective physical disease would be beneficial. The psychiatrist also told Misty in a gentle manner that, in order for him to help her, he had to keep their relationship at a formal, highly professional level.

The psychiatrist also explained the nature of Misty's personality and the nature of borderline personality disorder. He referred her to a female counselor who specialized in dialectical behavioral therapy (DBT), a psychotherapeutic approach for people with borderline personality disorder. The psychiatrist indicated that he would periodically see Misty for appointments, but that his role would be to oversee her treatment and continue to educate her about her diagnosis and treatment. Also, he would be able to interact with her other doctors and to help coordinate care.

Over the last five years, Misty's life has become less chaotic. She has been able to hold down a job and has developed several good friendships. She is currently dating a man who has a good job and is in recovery from alcoholism. He has been abstinent from alcohol for a decade. Each understands some of the demons that the other has had to face. Although their relationship has not been without fights and arguments, the two seem to be able to help each other. Misty's physical health has also stabilized. She has developed mild asthma as documented by appropriate lung tests, and these symptoms have responded well to the use of a steroid inhaler. She continues to see her counselor for periodic sessions or to discuss an occasional crisis. She checks in as well with her psychiatrist every four months to update him on how she is doing.

This case illustrates the following principles:

- The spectrum of disorders that is diagnosed as somatization disorder/borderline personality disorder has long-lasting symptoms and typically has initial manifestations during adolescence. These disorders can lead to marked dysfunction and disruption in a person's quality of life.

- If the psychiatric diagnoses go unrecognized, many unnecessary, and potentially harmful, medical procedures and treatments may be performed. Some medical diagnoses, just like some psychiatric diagnoses, are not well validated, meaning that the underlying cause is not understood and the diagnosis is not very helpful for describing the course of a patient's illness. Patients with somatization disorder are sometimes given impressive-sounding medical diagnoses by well-intentioned internists, but it is unclear whether these diagnoses have any explanatory power.

- The instability in mood associated with somatization disorder and borderline personality disorder can result in intentional medication overdoses (in this case with Tylenol), which can have severe medical consequences. Although Misty intended her overdose to be a "cry for help" and not an attempt to die, she was unaware that too much Tylenol could destroy her liver.

- Some well-meaning mental health professionals utilizing certain therapeutic techniques can make matters worse for suggestible patients, for example, by encouraging, usually inadvertently, the creation of false memories.

- Individuals with somatization disorder and borderline personality disorder have dramatic and complex psychiatric histories and can be very difficult to treat. Appropriate, limit-setting psychotherapeutic approaches can help decrease some of the chaotic behaviors. Psychiatric medications can sometimes be beneficial, but must be managed extremely carefully by a psychiatrist. The likelihood of medication overdoses is significant; the dramatic and volatile symptoms exhibited by these patients can also lead to inappropriate, but well-intentioned, use of multiple psychiatric medications (polypharmacy).

- Personality disorders can become less obtrusive as one reaches middle age, but they rarely go away completely. Efforts to minimize destructive behaviors and to encourage healthy behaviors "buy some time" and allow the natural history of this disorder (i.e., a gradual lessening of some of the symptoms over time) to help further. Certain forms of psychotherapy (e.g., DBT) can be very helpful in dealing with these disorders as well.

Case 4. Is Larry's Problem All about His Substance Abuse?

Larry started to smoke marijuana heavily during high school. When he was a freshman in college, he also started to drink heavily. Despite his abuse of these two substances, he was very bright and was able to finish his first two years of college successfully. Then, Larry started using cocaine. During the summer following his sophomore year, he began to experience psychotic symptoms. He heard God's voice telling him that he was born to save the world. His behavior changed dramatically. He started to preach in malls and to "cure people" by touching their shoulders. He talked rapidly, but sometimes his words didn't make much sense. He slept little. He bought a large car with money from his college fund and called it the "lordmobile." He didn't believe anything was wrong with him, and his parents were unable to convince him to see a doctor or go to an emergency room. Larry became very irritable and started to get into arguments with almost everyone he met. Some of these arguments became physical altercations. The police witnessed one such altercation and brought Larry to the local psychiatric hospital's emergency room.

In the emergency room, Larry was loud and belligerent. He punched one of the psychiatry technicians in the face. He refused admission and was committed to the hospital against his will for a 96-hour evaluation. During this time, Larry remained loud and belligerent, and he refused evaluation or medications. Because his behavior remained dangerous and he was unwilling to accept any type of help, the psychiatrist and hospital team decided that it was necessary to go through the judicial procedure to commit Larry for a longer period of hospitalization. Larry was assigned a lawyer who met with him in the hospital and accompanied him to the court hearing. The judge agreed with the doctors that Larry needed treatment and committed him to the hospital for another 21 days, during which time he could be treated with medications against his will.

Initially, Larry was treated with intramuscular injections of an antipsychotic medication. After three days, he agreed to take the medication orally. He started to be able to focus on conversations. The doctors told Larry that he likely was having a manic episode and that a mood stabilizer together with an antipsychotic medication would help him. In addition, the doctors said that the illicit drugs he had been taking may have contributed to his symptoms. Larry agreed to start taking lithium along with the antipsychotic medication. As he improved, he was taught more about bipolar disorder and the importance of avoiding marijuana, alcohol, and cocaine. The hospital team also worked with Larry's family, telling them that the use of all these substances would interfere with Larry's recovery. After two weeks, Larry was doing well and was discharged from the hospital with an appointment to see an outpatient psychiatrist in a week.

Larry did okay for several months. He returned to school. Unfortunately, he started to drink again and smoked both marijuana and cigarettes. He periodically forgot to take his medications for several days in a row. He gradually became more withdrawn and started to become convinced that the government was spying on him with special devices that could see through walls. He began to hear voices telling him to hide and not talk to anyone. He was concerned that his food was being poisoned, and he became suspicious that his roommates were part of a conspiracy. He barricaded himself in his college apartment bedroom. His roommates called his parents. Larry's dad and brother drove to the apartment and eventually had to take the door off its hinges in order to enter Larry's room. The room was a total mess. Larry had been using a corner of the room as a bathroom. He hadn't eaten or had anything to drink for several days.

Once again, Larry was hospitalized involuntarily, and once again, he was taken to court and committed for an additional 21 days. This time the doctors thought Larry's diagnosis was schizophrenia, and they continued prescribing an antipsychotic medication. Although he gradually improved, Larry didn't return to his earlier state of health. He came home after three weeks, but he remained suspicious and withdrawn. He said he was taking his antipsychotic medication, but this was hard to confirm. He was encouraged to go to a day hospital program, but he refused.

Larry was unable to go back to school. He found that he felt better smoking cigarettes and marijuana. He was able to give up his heavy drinking and stayed away from cocaine. Over the next several years, he had several psychotic episodes. It was difficult to tell whether his illness was bipolar disorder or schizophrenia or an illness that involves symptoms of both, called schizoaffective disorder. His behavior became so erratic and, at times, threatening that his family eventually felt it necessary to tell Larry to move out. Following his ninth hospitalization, his social worker helped Larry find a boarding home. There were eight other clients living there. Larry didn't know why he needed medications; he felt that cigarettes and marijuana helped him more than anything else. He also started using cocaine again, and unfortunately, he became dependent on it. He had no insight into the fact that he became significantly more disorganized and psychotic when he didn't take his medications and that the marijuana and cocaine made his behaviors worse.

For several years, Larry continued in this cycle of frequent hospitalizations, followed by short-term improvement of his psychotic symptoms and then by relapse associated with lack of compliance with medications and with use of illicit drugs. During one of his admissions, Larry agreed to be transferred to a 30-day inpatient substance abuse program. He kept taking his medications during this month-long program and was able to learn about problems associated with marijuana and cocaine. After the 30 days, he continued in an intensive day program and also became involved in a clubhouse rehabilitation program that taught job skills to people with severe mental illnesses such as schizophrenia or bipolar disorder. Larry discovered that he liked the idea of being able to work. The clubhouse staff was able to get Larry a job with a small company where he helped make and copy brochures. Larry's case manager worked closely with him and encouraged him to continue attending his drug abstinence-related group meetings and to keep his appointments with his psychiatrist. The case manager also helped Larry understand that he does much better when he avoids illicit drugs and alcohol and takes his medications. In fact, Larry agreed to take long-acting injections of his antipsychotic so that he wouldn't need to remember to take his pills.

Larry is now 40 years old. He continues to be treated with a long-acting antipsychotic medication, and his course has been complicated by a 50-pound weight gain and the development of type II diabetes mellitus. He receives care from an outpatient psychiatrist at the local hospital and from his primary care doctor for his diabetes. He continues to work and attend his group meetings. He still lives in a group home. He has learned to play guitar and enjoys music. He volunteers at the clubhouse, helping other clients to learn job skills. He isn't much of a people person and seems content with his job, boarding home, guitar, and television. He does exercise at the clubhouse several times a week.

He still finds that cigarettes help him concentrate, and so he hasn't given up smoking. His parents go out to supper with him about twice a month, and both they and Larry find these occasions meaningful.

This case illustrates the following principles:

- Sometimes, the nature of a psychotic illness can be easily diagnosed; at other times, distinguishing among bipolar disorder, schizoaffective disorder, schizophrenia, and a drug-induced psychotic state can be difficult. No laboratory tests help with this distinction, and the clinical course over time becomes one of the major determinants.

- Drugs of abuse can complicate both symptoms and treatment compliance. Some evidence suggests that some drugs of abuse can increase the risk for chronic psychotic illnesses. This is clearest for certain abused stimulant drugs, such as cocaine and amphetamines, but it is also true for marijuana, where specific genetic predis-positions coupled with marijuana use have been linked to schizophrenia.

- Eventually, recurrent psychotic illness can wear out the best-intentioned families. Families care, but they can do only so much for a patient before they burn out. There are community organizations that can be a big help for families in dealing with severe mental illnesses; the National Alliance on Mental Illness (NAMI) is one example.

- Psychotic illnesses can be very disabling. It is a sad fact that they are among the leading causes of disability in western countries. Furthermore, individuals with chronic psychotic disorders, such as schizophrenia, are more likely to die prematurely from a variety of causes, including suicide and cardiovascular disorders.

- Antipsychotic medication can be lifesaving for certain illnesses. Unfortunately, the medications have significant side effects, and in Larry's case, they contributed to his weight gain and diabetes. The continued use of an antipsychotic medication should trigger careful evaluation of the risk-benefit ratio, weighing side effects against the management of disabling and severe symptoms of psychosis.

- Treating substance abuse disorders can facilitate the successful treatment of psychotic disorders.

- Group support settings can be very important in the long-term care of patients with severe psychiatric illnesses. Job training as well as the social support provided by clubhouse rehabilitative approaches can be invaluable in helping individuals regain function.

Case 5. Why Is This 69-Year-Old Man Watching a Soccer Game No One Else Can See?

Mark had enjoyed a successful career as the chief executive officer of a small company, and he remained very active during retirement. He loved traveling with his wife Mary and visiting their grandkids. During the year prior to Mark's 69th birthday, his wife noticed that he wasn't as quick with numbers as he once was. He made some minor, careless errors with their investments and misplaced some important tax documents. He didn't remember recent conversations as well as he once did, but Mary thought this problem was related to the fact that he wasn't paying attention.

Six months before his birthday, Mark started to walk much more slowly. He had been an avid golfer all his life, but he seemed to take much longer getting ready for golf, and his golfing partners noticed that it took him forever to get in and out of the golf cart.

None of this was distressing. Mary thought that Mark's difficulties were simply due to his getting older. She did start to become more concerned, however, when she noticed Mark staring out the window a lot. When she asked what he was doing, he said he was watching kids playing soccer. There were no kids playing soccer. Mary became aware that Mark was having frequent visions that she couldn't see. He wasn't bothered by them, but Mary knew that his mind was playing tricks on him. She told him that she couldn't see what he saw, and he looked worried. She suggested that they tell his doctor about his visions, but he was embarrassed.

A few months later, Mary noticed that Mark would have periods during the day when he appeared confused. He would ask her the same question repeatedly or ask her the date or whether their son was home yet. Their son had his own family and lived in a different city. These episodes of confusion were discrete; that is, they would come and go. While they were occurring, they were obvious. They lasted about an hour, and then Mark would be back to normal.

Nonetheless, Mary became increasingly concerned and called their family physician. He suggested that they come in for an appointment. Mark needed to see the doctor for his annual checkup anyway and agreed to go. The doctor asked Mark about the visions, and Mark indicated that he didn't know why

Mary couldn't see the soccer games and wondered if something was wrong with her vision. The doctor checked Mark's memory by asking a brief series of questions and noticed that he wasn't as sharp as the doctor would have expected. On physical exam, the doctor noted that Mark was a bit stiff. His face looked much less expressive than in the past—almost like he had a poker face.

The doctor told Mark that there were some changes in his memory and that his mind might be making him see things that others were unable to see. He recommended that Mark see a psychiatrist at a nearby medical school who specialized in working with people over the age of 65. Mark reluctantly agreed to go. The geriatric psychiatrist reviewed the history with both Mark and Mary, including the results of Mark's recent annual checkup. The psychiatrist's examination of Mark included some brief cognitive testing (which included questions designed to test memory, thinking, and judgment) and psychiatric and neurologic exams. She also ordered a magnetic resonance imaging (MRI) brain scan, which showed only subtle changes in brain structure. The degree of these changes was not dramatic and not diagnostic of any particular disorder.

Still, considering all the available information, the psychiatrist determined that Mark was likely to have a mild form of a dementia known as "dementia with Lewy bodies" (DLB). She reviewed this diagnosis with both Mark and Mary and encouraged them to contact the local Alzheimer's Association. This group would be able to provide support and practical information about dementias, including DLB. The doctor prescribed a medication called Aricept (donepezil) to help slow the illness down and told them that this type of medicine had been shown to be about as helpful in DLB as in Alzheimer's dementia. Mary asked if there was a medication that could stop Mark's "visions." The doctor told her that people with DLB are very sensitive to the movement side effects of antipsychotic medications and suggested that Mark avoid using these medications unless the hallucinations became very frightening or disruptive. Furthermore, the benefit of antipsychotic medications for treating psychotic symptoms in the context of a dementia is not high. The psychiatrist encouraged Mark to continue with his activities and stressed the importance of pursuing heart-healthy behaviors, such as controlling his blood pressure and cholesterol levels and maintaining a good diet and a regular regimen of exercise.

Mark came back for a visit with the psychiatrist in six months. The illness had changed very little. He and Mary had traveled extensively. They had read more about dementias. They both were participating in groups run by the Alzheimer's Association. They also had met with a lawyer who had experience working with couples in which one of the spouses has an early dementia; the lawyer helped Mark and Mary to establish a living will and to plan for

Mark's likely deterioration in cognitive function. Mark told the psychiatrist that for the time being he felt fine. He realized that he had the ability to see things that Mary couldn't see, but he wasn't disturbed by these visions. Mary accepted that these visions were part of Mark's illness and didn't react when he was watching his "personal shows."

By the time Mark saw the psychiatrist a year later, he had experienced significant deterioration in both his memory and his movement disorder. He also had developed significant depressive symptoms. The psychiatrist explained that depression was common in this disorder and prescribed an antidepressant. Mark met with the psychiatrist for four sessions over the next two months, and his depressive symptoms improved substantially.

Over the next year, Mark's illness progressed significantly. He would leave the stove on after boiling water for tea. He was having trouble remembering conversations for more than a few minutes. He could no longer find his way around streets in his neighborhood. He walked slowly and occasionally lost his balance and fell. He was slow and stiff, his steps were small, and he had difficulty getting out of a chair without help. His mood was okay. He would stare off into space often and have broken conversations with people who weren't visible to others. Mark, Mary, and their family had learned that Mark's illness was associated with an accumulation of a protein called "synuclein," which is located in brain cells and involved in the formation of Lewy bodies, the likely cause of degeneration in Mark's brain. The entire family was participating in research at the medical school and hoped that their participation would help lead to a better understanding of this illness and, eventually, to a cure.

Three years after his initial symptoms, Mark died from pneumonia. The family honored his wishes for a brain autopsy, which showed Lewy bodies in several regions of the cerebral cortex.

This case illustrates the following principles:

- Some memory changes are normal with aging, and others are not. Psychiatrists, particularly those who specialize in working with elderly patients, can be helpful in making these distinctions.

- Visual hallucinations in an awake person are not normal and require medical and psychiatric evaluation.

- Hallucinations do not necessarily mean that a person has schizophrenia. Psychotic symptoms can occur in a variety of psychiatric, neurological, and medical disorders.

- Although Alzheimer's disease is the most common cause of dementia, clinical symptoms can help a physician differentiate Alzheimer's dementia from other dementias, including DLB.

- The use of different types of medications in treating dementias requires clinical expertise. For instance, in this example of DLB, Aricept might help delay the progression of the illness for a period of 6 to 12 months, and an antidepressant may help treat the co-occurring depression. However, antipsychotic medications can have severe side effects in persons with DLB. The risk-benefit ratio needs to be examined carefully.

- Brain autopsies are helpful in validating clinical diagnoses of dementia. This can be very important information for family members. In the meantime, research is rapidly progressing, and eventually clinicians will be able to diagnose with more certainty various forms of dementia during life. As we learn more about the clinical and neurochemical changes related to each dementia, treatments can eventually be developed that will slow down, stop, or perhaps even prevent the development or progression of symptoms.

Take-Home Messages

- Psychiatric disorders can occur at any age from early childhood to late adulthood. The age of onset can be very helpful in determining the nature of a disorder. For example, personality disorders usually have symptoms that begin in adolescence and rarely have their onset after age 25, unless the personality change occurs in the context of a head injury or other neurological condition. Dementias, on the other hand, can lead to marked changes in personality and other psychiatric symptoms but do not usually have their onset before age 50. Major depression can occur at any age.

- Psychiatric symptoms and syndromes have complex interactions with medical and neurological disorders. Among mental health professionals, psychiatrists have the most extensive training to deal with these complexities in diagnosis.

- Substance abuse can occur in some individuals as their primary (and only) psychiatric disorder. Often, however, substance abuse complicates other psychiatric disorders, contributing to major problems in treatment compliance, response to treatment, and long-term course of illness. It is extremely difficult to treat any psychiatric disorder occurring in the context of ongoing substance abuse.

• Psychiatric medications can be very helpful in dealing with psychiatric disorders. However, all medications have limitations and side effects. Psychotherapy, lifestyle interventions, and community support groups can play huge roles in helping patients and their families deal with the complex and at times devastating effects of psychiatric disorders.

··· *fourteen* ···

Trends in Psychiatry and Mental Health

A Brief Overview of Past Trends

Psychiatry has changed dramatically over the last several decades. Prior to the 1950s, psychoanalytic approaches dominated psychiatric thinking. These approaches were based on opinion and dogma and not empirical evidence. Examining the reliability or validity of psychoanalytic approaches in controlled clinical trials was not considered relevant. Psychoanalytic psychotherapy was considered an important, perhaps the most important, treatment modality. Such treatment usually required multiple therapy sessions per week conducted over extended periods of time, often years. When in the 1950s effective medications to treat mental disorders began to become available, many psychoanalysts felt that these medications could, at best, only cover up symptoms and that therapy was still required to help patients restructure their lives.

Then, during the 1960s and 1970s, faculty of Washington University's Department of Psychiatry helped to lead the field of psychiatry toward the medical model approach that we discussed previously in this book. A medical model approach encourages the use of empirical data from well-designed research studies to help define disorders and develop evidence-based treatments.

Research leads to knowledge, and knowledge leads to better understanding of illnesses and the development of better treatments. This scientifically based approach to studying and treating psychiatric disorders challenged the dogmatic approach of the psychoanalysts, and the psychiatric community initially did not look favorably upon the psychiatrists who developed this approach. This model has been the cornerstone of success in all medical disciplines, yet its initial implementation in psychiatry was considered heretical and odd.

One of the first consequences of the medical model was the development of more reliable definitions of illnesses based on specific diagnostic criteria. These definitions set the stage for studies showing that psychiatric disorders are very common. With this knowledge, academic psychiatrists and scientists in the pharmaceutical industry became interested in finding better treatments for specific disorders. The methodology for well-designed clinical trials developed, and increasing numbers of treatment studies were performed. Because neuroscience was advancing rapidly and new knowledge regarding brain chemistry, structure, and function was leading to a better understanding of how medications may influence brain and behavior, many of the early treatment studies involved medications. However, over time, other modalities, including various forms of psychotherapy, were studied in empirical clinical trials as well. This has provided the field with a sound basis for determining the most effective approaches for treating a given patient.

Interestingly, many of the medicines discovered to be helpful in patients with psychiatric disorders were found through serendipity (aka "luck"). For example, Thorazine (chlorpromazine) was developed originally to help people tolerate heart surgery; it was later observed to have calming effects on behavior, which led to clinical trials in patients with symptoms of schizophrenia. A medication called Tofranil (imipramine) was developed by chemically manipulating the structure of chlorpromazine in an attempt to develop another antipsychotic medication. However, Tofranil was found to have antidepressant rather than antipsychotic effects, and it became a mainstay of depression treatment. Because its chemical structure has three chemical rings, it is known as a "tricylic" antidepressant (TCA). Another example of serendipity is demonstrated in the discovery of monoamine oxidase inhibitor (MAOI) antidepressants. A medicine that was used to treat patients with tuberculosis also appeared to improve mood. The mechanism for this effect turned out to be the drug's influence on certain brain transmitter levels through inhibition of MAO, a protein that helps metabolize neurotransmitters such as serotonin, norepinephrine, and dopamine. These discoveries were occurring at the same time as research in brain neurochemistry was advancing, so the fields of psychopharmacology and neurochemistry grew up more or less hand-in-hand from the 1950s onward.

As a result of the effectiveness of early psychotropic medications, the treatment pendulum began to swing from psychodynamic therapy to pharmacological therapies. A mentality started to develop that psychiatric disorders were "chemical imbalances" and that medications could successfully treat these imbalances. Although this sounds good, the term *chemical imbalance,* as noted in Chapter 6, gives a false impression that we know what is actually going on in the brain. Obviously, major psychiatric disorders are related to imbalances of chemicals that regulate brain function, but this relationship really tells us nothing about the real causes of psychiatric disorders or about how medications actually produce their beneficial effects.

The advent of effective psychiatric medications led some people to believe that psychiatric treatment only required administering the correct pill or group of pills. These pills would then "cure" the illness or, at least, make a person remarkably better. This would be wonderful if it was true; unfortunately, it is not. Depending on the disorder, medications can clearly help, but not to the degree that many of us would like. Even when medications are helpful, they are often most helpful when used in combination with other forms of treatment, including talk therapies and lifestyle interventions. Recent large-scale studies of medication effectiveness, most notably the study called STAR*D (Sequenced Treatment Alternatives to Relieve Depression), have been sobering in this regard, indicating that remission of symptoms in major depression is achieved in only a subset of patients over a year of treatment. Contributors to the overall limited response rate include the complexities of major depression in many patients whose long-standing (chronic) symptoms, other coexisting medical and psychiatric disorders, and complicated life circumstances conspire to make treatment difficult. Similarly sobering results have been found in large-scale studies of schizophrenia (the Clinical Antipsychotic Trials of Intervention Effectiveness, or CATIE, study) and bipolar disorder (the Systematic Treatment Enhancement Program for Bipolar Disorder, or STEP-BD, study). In addition to the complexities of the illnesses themselves, part of the problem with poor response in all of these studies is that the current medications, while good, are just not good enough . . . yet.

Despite limitations, treatments are improving and are better than ever. The pendulum has clearly swung from a dogmatic psychoanalytic model to a medical model with an emphasis on careful diagnosis and a strong belief in the importance of research as the preferred way to advance the field. The sciences underlying psychiatry have advanced by leaps and bounds. It is both time-consuming and difficult to keep up with these advances. Pressures for simple solutions and aggressive marketing by the pharmaceutical industry have contributed to the impression that medications are magic bullets and may be all that is necessary to treat psychiatric disorders. Importantly for patients, such claims are more marketing than truth.

With this as background, let's now look at some of the current trends influencing the field of psychiatry. We will look especially at trends involving diagnosis, treatment, doctor–industry relationships, psychiatric education, and the mental health care workforce.

Trends in Diagnosis

The idea that psychiatric diagnoses can be reliable and valid (see Chapters 1 and 2) started to gain wide acceptance in the 1970s. The 1980 third edition of the *Diagnostic and Statistical Manual of Mental Disorders* (DSM-III) reflected these advances. Diagnostic criteria, when rigorously applied, allowed for a high degree of diagnostic agreement among different professionals. But diagnostic reliability doesn't mean that we understand the cause or mechanisms of a disorder. For instance, we can accurately differentiate schizophrenia from panic disorder, but we can't be certain whether the diagnostic criteria for each of these disorders accurately reflect specific biologic systems that are malfunctioning. Nevertheless, the standardized DSM terminology was tremendously helpful in jump-starting certain types of psychiatric research. In fact, over the last few decades, psychiatry has become one of the most intensely research-oriented fields in medicine, and rigorous methods in psychiatric studies are now the norm, putting psychiatry at the forefront of clinical studies across all fields of medicine.

Diagnosis, however, became a growth industry. DSM-IV, which was published in 1994, added a large number of "illnesses" that lacked substantial research supporting either their diagnostic reliability or their validity. Examples included certain personality disorders, some forms of post-traumatic stress disorder, and weakened versions of mood disorders. Why did this occur? The reasons are complex but include both scientific and political struggles within the field in which some factions pushed their own agendas ahead of empirical scientific rigor. Indeed, the DSM criteria for various disorders are achieved by consensus among leaders in the field with input from active clinicians. The criteria, however, are not written in stone, but rather are attempts to provide guidelines for making diagnoses. This fact has become somewhat lost these days, and diagnostic criteria have become reified and treated as gospel in some sectors. This has resulted in the DSM becoming the major resource for diagnostic definitions and diagnostic billing codes. In our opinion, this use of the DSM for payment decisions by the medical insurance industry has had an adverse effect on the clinical diagnoses that are actually used in the community. Physicians diagnose disorders that they are paid to treat. Third-party payers frown upon diagnostic uncertainty, even if that uncertainty reflects the truth for some cases. This forces mental health professionals to fit patients into categories that appear much neater than they actually are. This is a disturbing trend that significantly weakens the overall credibility of the field and may adversely affect the outcome of treatment.

Work is now well underway for the development of DSM-V. Is there really enough new information since the publication of DSM-IV to support launching an entirely new version of the DSM? Some, including we ourselves, would say there is not. Is it appropriate to publish a new DSM if there isn't enough scientific justification for this "new" diagnostic manual? This is debatable, but regardless, DSM-V will become a reality in the near future, and we will have to see how much of an advance it is over DSM-IV. One thing that is certain is that DSM-V will continue to make psychiatric diagnoses on the basis of clinical description and not objective tests. Laboratory studies will remain important only for determining whether other medical or neurological disorders are contributing to a clinical condition.

Eventually (and not in DSM-V), diagnoses will be rooted in etiology; that is, we will have a much better handle on both the biologic and genetic underpinnings of psychiatric illnesses and on their interaction with the environment. We may start to develop this depth of understanding for some psychiatric disorders during the next few decades. Although DSM-V may not represent a major leap forward, we predict that DSM-VI, when it is developed, could introduce us to a markedly different way of diagnosing and understanding psychiatric illnesses. At that point, we will likely be in a position to offer new and, it is hoped, mechanism-based treatments for mental disorders.

Trends in Treatments

As reviewed earlier in this chapter, treatments have moved away from dogmatic psychodynamic therapy and toward evidenced-based approaches. Current state-of-the-art treatment combines biologic, psychological, and social approaches—a so-called "biopsychosocial" approach to care. Much is being learned about various brain systems that are abnormal in different psychiatric illnesses. Such abnormalities may be triggered by environmental, psychosocial, or biologic stressors; sometimes, these abnormalities occur spontaneously. As the brain systems regulating emotions and thinking are better understood at anatomic, systems, and cellular levels, pharmacological treatment alternatives will likely increase. Some of these new treatments will probably be much more specific to particular illnesses than are current medications.

Knowledge in the field of genetics also is rapidly advancing, and it is likely that we soon will better understand an individual's predisposition to develop certain illnesses. This individualized approach to understanding risks for illness will be accompanied by the ability to predict an individual's response to specific treatments, including risks of certain side effects of treatments. Different biologic subtypes of illnesses may respond differently to particular treatments, and progress is being made in determining these specific subtypes. A nascent field with the unwieldy name of "psychiatric pharmacogenomics," which studies treatment response based on an individual's genetic heritage, in part reflects this progress in personalized medicine. In the future, genetics and neuroscience may lead us to entirely new ways of thinking about and categorizing psychiatric disorders, based much more on the inherent biology that is dysfunctional. In addition, variation in response to medications may depend on how an individual's body handles a particular drug. The ability to determine how an individual will physically handle a particular drug is already available for certain drugs.

During the next several decades, it is also likely that we will be able to use "nanotechnology" to deliver drugs attached to very small particles (called "nanoparticles") to very specific areas of the brain. As a hypothetical example, let's imagine that an illness is caused by a deficiency in a specific chemical in the amygdala, an area of the brain that is critical for processing emotions. Through nanotechnology, it may become possible to deliver a medication to restore the missing chemical directly to the amygdala. Such a drug delivery system could be highly advantageous and would likely avoid the side effects that occur as a result of the medication acting in other parts of the brain or body.

In the future, we also will better understand and appreciate specific psychological approaches. These approaches may utilize not just psychotherapies but perhaps specific activities designed to activate specific brain regions as well. For example, it is not hard to imagine that certain types of computer activities may target specific brain circuitry. Perhaps programs designed to teach people to better recognize various facial expressions may enhance a person's ability to become more empathetic and connected to others. Similarly, certain activities may help us better control our emotions. Some psychiatrists, such as C. Robert Cloninger, are already championing these concepts with what Cloninger refers to as "gymnasiums of the mind." While early in concept, these approaches are worthy of consideration and systematic empirical research.

Some of this may sound like science fiction. We don't believe it is. Neuroscientists already are working on ways to engineer proteins that can turn activity on and off in specific regions of the brain. For example, some psychiatric scientists, such as Karl Deisseroth at Stanford University, are engineering brain cells to express specific proteins (called "ion channels") that can be turned on or off with specific wavelengths of visible light. These proteins can be introduced into living animals and provide powerful ways to change function in very discrete areas of the brain—with a localized flash of the right type of light. Similarly, new chemicals are being developed that can be turned off and on in specific regions of the brain. Examples include certain novel neurosteroid molecules that normally are not active on their own but become active when exposed to certain wavelengths of visible light. The importance of these efforts is highlighted further by work we've mentioned previously—that of Helen Mayberg and colleagues at Emory University who are already using focal deep brain electrical stimulation to help patients with refractory and debilitating depression. The proof in concept for this idea comes from the field of neurology, where deep brain stimulation is now an accepted and useful form of treatment for some patients with severe Parkinson's disease.

Trends in the Relationships between Psychiatry and Industry

True scientific relationships between academia and industry (the pharmaceutical industry and the medical device industry, specifically) can be productive, important, and beneficial to society. Since the late 1990s, however, it has become evident that certain types of financial ties between physicians and industry that are primarily directed toward drug marketing are not in society's best interest. Because psychiatric drugs are among the most financially profitable products sold by the pharmaceutical industry, it is understandable that drug companies want doctors to prescribe their products. But the means by which these companies have pushed their agenda have exceeded the bounds of acceptable practice. Over the years, the pharmaceutical industry has provided physicians with numerous gifts ranging from inexpensive pens and trinkets to expensive and lavish trips. Offering physicians dinners at expensive restaurants to hear industry-paid speakers extol the benefits of a company's products has been very common. The practice of pharmaceutical representatives bringing gifts and food to doctors' offices has been, and is still, common. The business of advertising and influence is a core part of capitalism, but these practices have become excessive, and many physicians have been susceptible to them.

In addition, there are academic and clinical leaders in psychiatry who have close ties to the pharmaceutical industry. They can quite easily earn tens of thousands of dollars a year (and, in some cases, hundreds of thousands of dollars) by giving talks to other doctors about a company's products. Others earn substantial amounts by consulting for and advising companies about product development. It's interesting that many physicians think that these financial relationships between doctors and industry may influence others but have no influence on their own thinking. One would hope that psychiatrists would know better, but many don't. In fact, although these practices occur in every branch of medicine, psychiatry may be one of the most problematic disciplines in medicine in terms of conflicted relationships with industry.

We mentioned in Chapter 12 that top medical centers have now started to implement policies to minimize the conflicts of interest that can exist when academic faculty have nonscientific relationships with industry. For instance, at Washington University in St. Louis, there are now strict policies regulating financial interactions between faculty and industry. Each clinician and each researcher is required to disclose financial relationships to a conflict-of-interest committee. If this independent review committee determines that the reported relationships have the potential to influence research or clinical care, a management strategy is implemented to minimize or eliminate the conflict. Sometimes, faculty members are required to disclose their conflicts to research participants, patients, and journals; at other times, faculty must surrender their financial interests if they wish to continue their research or clinical practice. Similar policies have been implemented at many medical centers and are sensitizing academic leaders to the important responsibility they have in remaining unbiased by financial considerations when advancing the field of medicine through research, teaching, and clinical care.

Many medical schools also have set strict limitations on the interactions of pharmaceutical representatives with their personnel. For example, at our university, no gifts to personnel of any type are allowed. Drug representatives may not interact with medical students or residents unless supervised by faculty. Drug company representatives must have appointments to see individual faculty members; they can't just drop in for a visit. "Free lunches" provided by drug companies are not permitted.

Similarly, academic institutions themselves have conflicts of interest, including conflicts that involve the pharmaceutical and medical device industries. Academic medical centers play key roles in influencing the direction of research and health care. Such centers, although not-for-profit, can have substantial financial impact at both local and national levels. Academic institutions often receive financial support from donors, including donations from various industries. It is important that such financial support be carefully reviewed in order to manage any potential conflicts of interest that may occur if the support is accepted. Thus, another recent trend is for these institutions to establish policies and committees to oversee institutional conflicts of interest. Such reviews are in addition to the reviews of individual faculty members. Again, this is a trend that is extremely healthy for faculty, research subjects, and patients.

The trend to separate physicians from the financial influence of industry is being most aggressively pursued in medical school settings; they are training centers and the home of the field's thought leaders. But this trend has not yet reached into the realm of private practice. Perhaps policies will soon be implemented by medical organizations that will diminish the influence of industry on individual physicians in practice settings because this influence is known to affect physicians' choices of medications and recommendations. Interestingly, one of the arguments we often hear in defense of the importance of exposure to drug company representatives during medical school and residency training is that doctors need to be prepared to interact with these salespersons once they enter practice. Our response to this argument is "why?" Students and residents are taught to evaluate new products scientifically and impartially as part of their training. If physicians need to meet with drug company representatives (who have limited scientific and usually no clinical training) in order to learn about new products, then our medical training system is failing and needs to be revamped.

The bottom line regarding this issue is that doctors are increasingly regulating themselves. They must do so, and they must do so effectively. If they don't, doctors will be regulated by outside forces, much like what has already occurred with Medicare where a third-party payer dictates the type of information that must appear in a medical record. Some states are beginning to require pharmaceutical companies to list the details of their financial relationships with individual doctors. Documentation about such relationships will likely become easily available on the Internet. If faced with this risk of public embarrassment, resulting in patients knowing how much money their own doctors are accepting from companies whose drugs they recommend to their patients, perhaps those physicians will change their habits.

It is our strong belief that the great majority of psychiatrists and mental health professionals truly care about their patients and make their patients' interests their top priority. But big business has become an increasing influence on all aspects of medicine during the last several decades. Major academic centers are leading the way to remind all doctors that their primary responsibilities are to patients and society, not to themselves. This trend of sensitizing physicians to these issues is healthy. In our opinion, patients must be sensitized to these issues as well. As we've emphasized previously, patients have a right to know about the potential conflicts their doctors may have and to have an informed conversation with their doctors about these issues. Conflicts of interest can and will influence the type of care that is delivered.

Trends in Psychiatric Education

In Chapter 4, we described the residency training that psychiatrists receive after they finish medical school. This training lasts four years for general psychiatrists; subspeciality training—for example, in child and adolescent psychiatry—may take another one or two years to complete. Several interesting and important trends are occurring in psychiatric education at the level of residency training. We will highlight a few of these trends here.

Accredited residency programs in all fields of medicine are certified by a national organization, the Accreditation Council for Graduate Medical Education (ACGME). Since the 1990s, ACGME has developed a new approach to resident education based on the achievement of competency in six specified areas. Residency programs are expected to construct their curriculum around these six areas, and all trainees are expected to achieve competency in all six areas by the time they graduate and enter into unsupervised practice settings. The first two competency areas deal with attaining an adequate knowledge base of medical information and learning how to apply this information to the care of patients. The formal titles of these two competencies are Medical Knowledge and Patient Care, respectively. The third area deals with competency in Interpersonal and Communication Skills, highlighting the important skills that doctors must have to interact effectively with patients, families, and other health care professionals. The fourth competency is Practice-based Learning and Improvement. This competency stresses continuous self-improvement through a review of the physician's own practice and efforts to keep up to date with changes in the field. Professionalism is the fifth competency area—that is, the importance of understanding the duties and obligations of being a doctor and of behaving in a professional manner as one assumes the demanding responsibilities of this profession. The sixth and final competency area is called Systems-based Practice. This area deals with learning how to work effectively with other health care professionals to coordinate excellent patient care within different health care delivery systems. As the field of medicine evolves, it is likely that the systems of care delivery will change. Preparing physicians to understand, lead, and adapt to this evolution while maintaining high-quality patient care is critically important.

Advances in all fields of medicine are moving at an incredible pace, and thus continuing medical education (CME) to keep up with these advances is essential. States generally require physicians to participate in CME in order to renew their licenses, and the American Board of Psychiatry and Neurology (ABPN), similar to boards in other fields of medicine, requires that psychiatrists participate in continuous learning activities in order to maintain their board certification. A recertification exam occurs every ten years, and during that ten-year interval, maintenance-of-certification exercises are required. These exercises involve rigorous educational activities and self-evaluation.

Finally, residency programs continuously evaluate their curriculum and the type of medical knowledge that should be taught during residency training. Four years is really not that long of a time in which to teach trainees what they need to know about psychiatry in addition to the six general medical competency areas just mentioned. Residents work up to 80 hours per week in the hospital; this does not include the time they spend reading and studying on their own. Psychiatry is a broad field. Multiple scientific disciplines form the knowledge base for the field and include neurobiology (across many levels ranging from molecular to systems and cognitive neuroscience), genetics, epidemiology, evolutionary sciences, cross-cultural sciences, psychology, neurology, and general medicine. The current trend is to teach a core base of knowledge that prepares trainees for the various certifying exams that they will be taking. Beyond that, different training programs emphasize different areas of this broad knowledge base in psychiatry and may utilize different teaching techniques to impart the information believed to be most important for tomorrow's psychiatry. Are some schools teaching tomorrow's psychiatry in a better fashion than other schools? There is no way of really knowing, but we believe that the best programs emphasize diverse training beyond the basic core competencies to prepare the next generation of psychiatrists for rapidly changing scientific and clinical landscapes.

Trends in Demographics and Health Care Delivery

Recent projections indicate that there is a substantial and increasing doctor shortage in the United States. Medical schools are being encouraged to train more doctors, but that may not translate into an increase in the number of positions that are available in post-medical school residency training programs. Thus, simply increasing the number of medical students may not improve access to well-trained physicians. This is because residency training is expensive, and the US Balanced Budget Act of 1997 placed significant caps on federal funding to institutions for post-medical school trainees in all disciplines. Unless nonfederal sources of funding are identified to support residency training positions, academic institutions cannot simply offer more training slots to medical school graduates. In fact, under current mandates, for one specialty to increase its number of training positions, another program must give up some of its positions. This is called a "zero-sum game" in economics and does not lead to an overall increase in well-trained physicians.

There are some specialties where the doctor shortage is significantly greater than it is in others. Psychiatry is one such "shortage specialty," and the shortage in child psychiatry is particularly critical. This situation will become even more noticeable in the near future because the average age of psychiatrists is older than the average age of doctors in many other fields and therefore more psychiatrists are closer to retirement. A large influx of individuals entered psychiatry following World War II and through the 1960s, but that increase was not sustained in subsequent decades. Thus, as those psychiatrists age and reach retirement, they are not being replaced at an equal rate by new psychiatrists. At the same time, the mental health needs of specific populations are likely to grow. As the elderly population increases, for example, so too will the psychiatric and neuropsychiatric illnesses that are common and complex in this population. Moreover, psychiatric disorders have recently been recognized by the World Health Organization (WHO) as some of the most disabling illnesses worldwide. In light of these indications of increased need for psychiatric expertise, it is unfortunate that we are faced with a major shortage of psychiatrists.

There are of course many other professionals who have various levels of training in mental health care, including clinical psychologists, social workers, and licensed counselors, and they provide specialized and needed expertise, including administering psychotherapies, incorporating social interventions, and determining other available resources and support systems for patients. In some states, stop-gap attempts to deal with the psychiatrist shortage are being considered, including giving psychologists and other nonmedical professionals the ability to prescribe psychotropic medications. As we noted earlier in the book, we believe this trend is extremely disturbing and dangerous because these nonphysician professionals, while good at what they are trained to do, have no training in medicine and are not equipped to deal with the complexities of concurrent medical illnesses, medication side effects, and interactions among medications. Patients are very likely to suffer as a result, and malpractice attorneys may be the only real beneficiaries of these "solutions" to the shortage of psychiatrists. Primary care doctors do, however, have the expertise (i.e., medical school training) to manage medications as part of a team approach. Psychiatrists can help oversee treatments and advise the primary care doctor about medical/psychiatric issues.

Ultimately, the most compelling trend is this: The ability of different members of the mental health care delivery team to work together and with members of the general medical health care team is essential now and will become increasingly so in the future if we are to deliver adequate care to our population. These team approaches will likely take advantage of the revolution in electronic and video communications. Flexibility of delivery systems will become essential. For instance, when a family doctor needs an informal consultation with a psychiatrist, this should be possible with video conferencing. Efficiency with improved quality will be the challenge. It will be critical that professionals across a wide range of disciplines work together to bring about a general health care delivery system that is of high quality, flexible, and affordable, and that takes advantage of each professional's specific training and talent. The development and funding of such a system are, however, some of the major political challenges facing our country today.

Take-Home Messages

- The field of psychiatry has changed dramatically since the 1960s. Evidence-based medical model approaches are now the standards in the field.

- The field will continue to change dramatically in the future. Psychiatric education must equip practitioners with the skills required to keep up with rapidly advancing scientific changes. Other current trends related to these changes involve diagnosis, treatment, financial relationships with industry, and demographics.

- These trends affect consumers because they influence psychiatric practice and ultimately the quality of mental health care delivery.

$\cdots$ *fifteen* $\cdots$

The Future of Psychiatry:
Reasons for Optimism

This is an exciting time in psychiatry. In some ways, psychiatry in the early 21st century can be compared to fields like physics and genetics at the turn of the 20th century. At that time, physics was embarking on a magical transformation, and new ideas and methods were developing rapidly. An enormous expansion in knowledge about the nature of atoms led later in the century to the development of nuclear power and other advances. Scientists like Einstein, Heisenberg, and Bohr became household names, and terms like *nuclear*, *relativity*, and *uncertainty* became part of our common vocabulary. In the early 1900s, the potential for the field of genetics could not even be imagined. The manipulation of genes and the sequencing of more than 3 billion building blocks in the human genome were unthinkable goals even in the 1970s, and yet they have now been achieved. We believe that the scientific knowledge of the human brain is currently in a similar position. Over the next 50 to 100 years, neuroscience research will lead scientists to understand in exquisite detail how humans process information, express and regulate emotions, and motivate themselves to achieve specific goals. This information will affect many clinical and scientific disciplines, including neurology, psychology, biomedical engineering, and computer sciences, but it will likely pay its greatest dividends in psychiatry. Interdisciplinary studies involving genetics, cognitive psychology, neuroimaging, and cellular and systems neuroscience offer great hope for understanding the mechanisms that contribute to psychiatric dysfunction and for finding new and innovative ways to treat mental illnesses.

We further believe that this new information will help elucidate the evolution of the human nervous system and the factors that make the human brain unique. It is already clear that the enhanced functions of the human brain do not necessarily reflect a larger genome than other species; current research suggests that humans have about 25,000 genes, which is not many more than the genes that fruit flies or worms have and not even as many as some plants have. Rather, it is the ability of our genes to adapt rapidly by turning on or off in response to events in the environment and by producing alternative proteins based on how genes are spliced together that may have allowed us to develop relatively sophisticated levels of intellectual, emotional, and motivational skills. Even greater opportunities for understanding the products and functions expressed by our genes are offered by the emerging field of epigenetics, which studies heritable factors that are not strictly encoded in the human genome but are the result of chemical modifications of DNA or proteins associated with DNA that can occur in response to environmental factors. Similarly, the emerging fields of proteomics (studying how proteins function), lipidomics (how fats and fat-derived messengers work), and systems biology will complement work in genomics to produce a more coherent picture of how neural systems operate. In this chapter, we will highlight a few other areas where we think science is generating optimism for the field of psychiatry.

The Brain Is Plastic

A recurring theme in this book is that humans are capable of learning, and they can adapt to extremely difficult environments. These simple statements are important truisms. If these statements were not true, humans would not have evolved as a species or survived the harshness of planet Earth or even competition with other animals, including other humans. The fact that humans still exist and have expanded their influence on the planet is a great tribute to our ability to adapt despite our being neither the fastest nor the strongest of animals. The ability of humans to learn, remember, and adapt is directly related to the changeableness (plasticity) of the human brain. Whenever we learn new information, the connections between nerve cells in the brain are modified. The activity of some connections (called synapses) increases, while the activity of other synapses decreases. The initial changes involve local chemical alterations in the way synapses transmit and receive information from other neurons. These initial chemical changes eventually lead to structural changes in the brain; that is, more connections and more complex connections form. The longer lasting of these changes require the turning on and turning off of specific genes; therefore, learning involves gene expression. Changes in synaptic connections represent a major way by which memories are formed. But as we all know, some memories fade, and it is likely that newly formed connections must be reinforced by ongoing brain activity in order for these connections to survive. The important points to remember are that learning alters the actual structure of the brain and that genes are involved in learning.

Although neurons and synapses located in many areas of the brain are capable of the changes involved in learning and memory, the amount of structural tailoring that actually occurs varies among different types of neurons and regions of the brain. As noted before, one brain region that plays an absolutely critical role in the formation of new memories is the hippocampus, a region that also appears to be very important in several major psychiatric disorders. The hippocampus receives inputs from all over the nervous system and helps to bind pieces of information together, allowing us to form complex associations between events that happen and the timing and location of these events. Importantly, the hippocampus is a short-term storage device. For longer-term storage of memories, information must be passed on to the larger neocortex where it is available for later recall. The way all this happens is increasingly being understood at molecular, structural, and systems levels. Many scientists have contributed to these efforts, but perhaps none has done more to advance the field than Nobel laureate, neuroscientist, and psychiatrist Eric Kandel. Starting with his studies of the simple nervous system in the sea snail, *Aplysia californica*, Kandel and his colleagues helped to explain in exquisite detail how animals learn and how learning influences behavior. This learning has been investigated not only in the context of responses to adverse circumstances (like tail shocks in *Aplysia* or fear conditioning in rodents), but also, more recently, in the way rodents learn to negotiate different spaces and even how animals learn "safety" signals when they are in an environment where harm will not come to them.

We believe that the importance of this work to psychiatry is obvious. In effect, memories are a large component of what it means to be human and who we are as individuals. What may be less clear is that brain plasticity is really what psychiatric treatment is all about. Whether it is through the use of medications or electroconvulsive therapy (ECT) to treat severe depression and psychosis or the use of psychotherapy to treat anxiety disorders and depression, the therapeutic approaches in psychiatry all work via changes in the brain that lead to benefits. If the brain were not plastic, patients with psychiatric disorders would have no hope for improvement or recovery.

Rather, the advances in psychiatric treatments over the last half of the 20th century reflect the ability of treatments to influence brain function in a positive way. We believe that psychiatrists will increasingly have to become expert at understanding brain plasticity and learn how to exploit this plasticity for therapeutic purposes. Hence, treatment for psychiatric disorders will be strongly influenced by advances in the arena of synaptic biology, including an increasing understanding about how the brain develops as it matures. In fact, work by innovative psychiatrists such as Kerry Ressler at Emory University and others is already pointing the way to new strategies to extinguish fear-based learning, and these are leading to clinical trials of new ways to treat certain psychiatric disorders.

Neurogenesis and Psychiatry

The story about neurogenesis (the formation of new nerve cells in the adult brain) is really part of the larger story about brain plasticity. Put another way, neurogenesis reflects the amazing resilience and plasticity of our brains. Expanding upon observations initially made years ago about birds, it has become clear that certain parts of the human brain are capable of generating new neurons throughout life, even during old age. Not all regions of the brain appear to have this ability to grow new nerve cells, but two regions, the dentate gyrus of the hippocampus and areas near the lateral ventricles in the olfactory system (which is involved in the sense of smell), are really good at it. The dentate gyrus plays a key role in the function of the hippocampus, the region that is so critical for memory processing. It is likely that a thousand or more new neurons are born in this region each day and can be incorporated into the circuitry of the hippocampus where they help enhance certain types of learning. These new neurons may be particularly important for processing new information.

Why is this important for psychiatry? Some things are good for neurogenesis, and other things are bad. Stress and stress hormones (like cortisol) have bad effects on neurogenesis. Alcohol and probably other drugs of abuse also interfere with either new cell formation or healthy connections between cells. The effect of other disorders on neurogenesis is less clear, but there is reasonable evidence to suggest that several major psychiatric disorders, such as major depression and schizophrenia, are associated with shrinkage or loss of cells in parts of the brain, particularly the hippocampus, and the exact relationships among illness, stress, and shrinkage of brain cells are areas of active investigation. Some treatments, such as lithium, may actually help to protect neurons from a variety of insults by inhibiting chemical pathways that lead to cell damage. Antidepressants work differently than lithium, but they may also help to protect certain types of brain cells. Additionally, lithium, antidepressant medications, and other treatments for depression, such as ECT, appear to augment neurogenesis in the dentate gyrus.

Certain lifestyle interventions can also promote neurogenesis. As discussed earlier in the book, some of these lifestyle activities (e.g., exercise and calorie restriction or weight loss, assuming one is overweight) enhance new nerve-cell formation or growth and are good for both physical and mental health. Learning and environmental enrichment, which refers to living in complex and challenging, but not overly stressful, situations, also enhance neurogenesis and thereby promote brain health. Psychotherapies are forms of complex learning, and thus it is very likely that certain psychotherapies enhance the generation of new neurons in the adult brain. It has also been shown that "exercising the brain" with puzzles, games, and social activities is good for the aging brain and may be a way that people can maintain their cognitive function as they age.

It remains uncertain whether neurogenesis represents a critical component of the therapeutic benefits in psychiatric treatments. However, at least two independent groups of scientists have found that inhibiting neurogenesis prevents at least some of the effects of antidepressants in rodents. Furthermore, the production of new neurons in the dentate gyrus may be important in correcting some of the dysfunction in hippocampal-prefrontal cortex neurocircuitry that appears to be involved in illnesses such as depression. It makes sense that the ability to grow new nerve cells in specific brain regions may have therapeutic potential. More therapeutic options will be developed as scientists learn how to successfully stimulate the birth of new nerve cells in specific brain regions. Neurogenesis could therefore prove to be a real "growth area" for psychiatry.

Science Will Win

One of the strongest reasons we are optimistic about the future of psychiatry is the recent rate of progress in all of biomedical research. We have alluded to the major advances in genetics, molecular biology, neurobiology, and cognitive sciences that have taken place since the late 1980s. Psychiatry is especially well positioned to take advantage of these advances and to build on them. If we learned anything during the 20th century, it is that the capabilities of research involving both fundamental basic science and applied technologies have been amazing. Now, in the early 21st century, scientists have the ability to do things that were unimaginable even 30 years ago. We have made tremendous progress in gene sequencing, molecular biology, membrane and receptor biophysics, synaptic and systems biology, and neuroimaging. While it is unclear whether advances will continue at the current pace, one only has to look at developments in such fields as computer science to see how rapidly things can change. Consider how fast new computer technologies have replaced older ones and how quickly and often computing capability has doubled. Our laptops today make even the most sophisticated computers of the 1970s look like dinosaurs.

It is now possible to envision studies that will allow us to test very specific hypotheses about how humans process information, including social and emotional information. There are already excellent models for studying various forms of learning and memory in nonhuman species. Using known analogies to the human brain, it is possible to extend these studies to human learning. Based on a better understanding of fundamental emotional behaviors in animals through the work of many scientists such as Jaak Panksepp, Joseph LeDoux, Michael Meaney, Eric Nestler, and others, it may be possible to develop animal models for studying primary emotional systems and their development in the brain. Investigators have already created some animal models to study social dominance and social defeat, and these models are likely to prove useful for understanding how emotional circuitry goes awry under stressful conditions. This work could be highly relevant to understanding mood and anxiety disorders.

Progress in cognitive and psychiatric sciences is generating tremendous enthusiasm among scientists who do not consider themselves to be psychiatric researchers. Animal models used to study specific genetic defects underlying certain forms of mental retardation in humans—disorders such as Fragile X syndrome (the most common heritable form of mental retardation), Williams syndrome, and others—are providing information that is leading to new optimism that prevention and treatment of these disorders are possible. These types of advances are making psychiatry much more attractive to a new generation of clinician-scientists, particularly those with combined MD and PhD degrees. These individuals are trained in both fundamental biology and clinical science and represent many of the best and brightest of today's medical students. Based on our experience at Washington University in St. Louis, an increasing number of these individuals may be choosing psychiatry as their career path. These individuals bring the hope of new ideas and new scientific methods to psychiatric science. Bright young scientists are the lifeblood of any scientific discipline, and this influx of talented, well-trained physician-scientists speaks extremely well for the future of the science of psychiatry.

New Vistas in Diagnosis and Treatment

Future progress in psychiatry will require better ways to diagnose and validate psychiatric disorders. As noted earlier in this book, validation remains a significant challenge and is currently based on clinical observation and the longitudinal course of the disorders. Validation based on genetics, brain mechanisms, and objective laboratory tests is lacking. We are at least beginning, however, to gain an understanding of the biological and genetic basis of psychiatric illnesses. Achieving a full grasp of these dimensions may take a good portion of the next century to become a reality for most psychiatric disorders, but there's no question that it will be realized. We are already approaching this level of sophistication in our understanding of some neuropsychiatric illnesses, such as Alzheimer's disease. In many ways, advances in the research on Alzheimer's disease represent a model for what may be possible with other major neuropsychiatric disorders. Detailed information about the pathological changes underlying this dementia, including information about the regions of the brain affected earliest and most intensely, are leading to better insights into not only possible mechanism-based therapies but also the ways in which our brains process information.

In psychiatry, we applaud the efforts to use sophisticated neuroimaging to study how humans make cognitive and emotional decisions, direct and focus attention, and interact with each other while playing certain types of complex social games. We believe these types of studies will pay huge dividends in helping us to understand normal and abnormal function of the brain. In these latter efforts, creative scientists such as Marc Raichle, Jonathan Cohen, Read Montague, Steve Peterson, and others are leading the way.

Today, it is easy to envision a future where psychiatric diagnosis is based on understanding fundamental defects in thinking, emotional processing, and motivational systems. In such a world, our traditional categories of psychotic disorders, mood disorders, anxiety disorders, cognitive disorders, and even personality disorders may need to be completely revised. In such a world, treatments might be much more based on underlying mechanisms, and there might be enhanced opportunities for early identification and even prevention of the disorders. In addition to the work on dementias, current research on the biology of syndromes associated with mental retardation is a great example of the potential opportunities.

In our view, psychiatry remains the most "human" of all medical disciplines. It deals with the problems that make us most human—the things that define our minds and our selves. Today, good psychiatric practice demands close attention to the doctor–patient relationship, a relationship that is built on meaningful and highly professional interpersonal interactions. Even in a future world where advances in neuroscientific research expand available treatment options for psychiatric disorders, humans will remain social beings. Therefore, understanding the psychology and social aspects of patients always will remain important to the therapeutic process. Furthermore, the quality of the doctor–patient relationship will remain a critical factor in the success of psychiatric treatment. This aspect of our field should never change. The doctor–patient relationship can only be enhanced when doctors are able to offer their patients better explanations for the mechanisms behind their psychiatric disorders and to recommend more and better treatment options. This will come from the eventual triumph of broadly conceptualized neuroscience.

Bibliography

Books for the Consumer

Andreasen, N. C. (2005). *The creating brain: The neuroscience of genius*. New York: Dana Press.

Angell, M. (2004). *The truth about the drug companies: How they deceive us and what to do about it*. New York: Random House.

Axelrod, R. (1984). *The evolution of cooperation*. Cambridge, MA: Basic Books.

Barabási, A.-L. (2002). *Linked: The new science of networks*. Cambridge, MA: Perseus Publishing.

Bok, D. (2003). *Universities in the marketplace: The commercialization of higher education*. Princeton, NJ: Princeton University Press.

Burns, D. D. (1980). *Feeling good: The new mood therapy*. New York: William Morrow & Co.

Cloninger, C. R. (2004). *Feeling good: The science of well-being*. New York: Oxford University Press.

Damasio, A. (1999). *The feeling of what happens: Body and emotion in the making of consciousness*. San Diego, CA: Harcourt.

Dukakis, K., & Tye, L. (2006). *Shock: The healing power of electroconvulsive therapy*. New York: Avery.

Edelman, G. M. (2004). *Wider than the sky: The phenomenal gift of consciousness*. New Haven, CT: Yale University Press.

Fulgham, R. (1996). *All I really need to know I learned in kindergarten: Uncommon thoughts on common things*. New York: Fawcett Columbine.

Gazzaniga, M. S. (2005). *The ethical brain: The science of our moral dilemmas*. New York: Dana Press.

Goldberg, E. (2001). *The executive brain: Frontal lobes and the civilized mind*. New York: Oxford University Press.

Hawkins, J. (with Blakeslee, S.). (2004). *On intelligence*. New York: Times Books.

Kandel, E. R. (2006). *In search of memory: The emergence of a new science of mind*. New York: WW Norton & Company.

Kassirer, J. P. (2005). *On the take: How medicine's complicity with big business can endanger your health*. New York: Oxford University Press.

LeDoux, J. (2002). *Synaptic self: How our brains become who we are*. New York: Viking Press.

Linden, D. J. (2007). *The accidental mind: How brain evolution has given us love, memory, dreams, and God*. Cambridge, MA: Belknap Press.

Minsky, M. (2006). *The emotion machine: Commonsense thinking, artificial intelligence, and the future of the human mind*. New York: Simon & Schuster.

Montague, R. (2006). *Why choose this book? How we make decisions*. New York: Dutton Press.

Quartz, S. R., & Sejnowski, T. J. (2002). *Liars, lovers and heroes: What the new brain science reveals about how we become who we are*. New York: William Morrow.

Ramachandran, V. S. (2004). *A brief tour of human consciousness: From impostor poodles to purple numbers*. New York: Pi Press.

Ramachandran, V. S., & Blakeslee, S. (1998). *Phantoms in the brain: Probing the mysteries of the human mind*. New York: William Morrow.

Ridley, M. (2003). *Nature via nurture: Genes, experience, and what makes us human*. New York: HarperCollins Publishers.

Schacter, D. L. (2001). *The seven sins of memory: How the mind forgets and remembers.* Boston: Houghton Mifflin.

Watts, D. J. (2003). *Six degrees: The science of a connected age.* New York: WW Norton & Company.

Textbooks and Manuals

Abrams, R. (2002). *Electroconvulsive therapy* (fourth edition). New York: Oxford University Press.

American Psychiatric Association. (1994). *Diagnostic and statistical manual of mental disorders* (fourth edition). Washington, DC: American Psychiatric Association.

American Psychiatric Association. (2006). *American Psychiatric Association practice guidelines for the treatment of psychiatric disorders. Compendium 2006.* Arlington, VA: American Psychiatric Association.

Beck, A. T., Rush, A. J., Shaw, B. F., & Emery, G. (1979). *Cognitive therapy of depression.* New York: The Guilford Press.

Goldsmith, S. K., Pellman, T. C., Kleinman, A. M., & Bunney, W. E. (Eds.) (2002). *Reducing suicide: A national imperative.* Washington, DC: National Academies Press.

Goodwin, D. W., & Guze, S. B. (1996). *Psychiatric diagnosis* (fifth edition). New York: Oxford University Press.

Guze, S. B. (1992). *Why psychiatry is a branch of medicine.* New York: Oxford University Press.

Guze, S. B. (Ed.). (1997). *Washington University adult psychiatry.* St. Louis, MO: Mosby.

Hales, R. E., Yudofsky, S. C., & Gabbard, G. O. (Eds.). (2008). *The American Psychiatric Publishing textbook of psychiatry* (fifth edition). Washington DC: American Psychiatric Publishing.

Lilienfeld, S. O., Lynn, S. J., & Lohr, J. M. (Eds.). (2003). *Science and pseudoscience in clinical psychology.* New York: The Guilford Press.

Meyer, R. E., & McLaughlin, C. J. (Eds.). (1998). *Between mind, brain, and managed care: The now and future world of academic psychiatry.* Washington, DC: American Psychiatric Press.

Morris, J. C., Galvin, J. E., & Holtzman, D. M. (Eds.). (2006). *Handbook of dementing illnesses* (second edition). New York: Taylor & Francis.

Panksepp, J. (2004). *Affective neuroscience: The foundations of human and animal emotions.* New York: Oxford University Press.

Robins, L. N., & Regier, D. A. (1991). *Psychiatric disorders in America: The Epidemiologic Catchment Area Study.* New York: Free Press.

Rubin, E. H., & Zorumski, C. F. (Eds.). (2005). *Adult psychiatry* (second edition). Malden, MA: Blackwell Publishing.

Sadock, B. J., & Sadock, V. A. & Ruiz, P. (Eds.). (2009). *Kaplan & Sadock's comprehensive textbook of psychiatry* (ninth edition). Philadelphia: Lippincott Williams & Wilkins.

Schatzberg, A. F., & Nemeroff, C. B. (Eds.). (2006). *Essentials of clinical psychopharmacology* (second edition). Washington, DC: American Psychiatric Publishing.

Srole, L., Sanger, T., Michael, S., Opler, M. K., & Rennie, T. A. C. (1962). *Mental health in the metropolis: The Midtown Manhattan Study.* New York: McGraw-Hill.

Weissman, M. M., Markowitz, J. C., & Klerman, G. L. (2000). *Comprehensive guide to interpersonal therapy.* New York: Basic Books.

Zorumski, C. F., & Rubin, E. H. (Eds.). (2005). *Psychopathology in the genome and neuroscience era.* Washington, DC: American Psychiatric Publishing.

Selected Books and Articles Organized by Topic

Psychiatric Diagnosis

American Psychiatric Association. (1994). *Diagnostic and statistical manual of mental disorders* (fourth edition). Washington, DC: American Psychiatric Association.

Andreasen, N. C. (1979). Thought, language and communication disorders. *Archives of General Psychiatry, 36,* 1315–1321.

Benton, T., Staab, J., & Evans, D. L. (2007). Medical co-morbidity in depressive disorders. *Annals of Clinical Psychiatry, 19,* 289–303.

Black, K.J., & Guze, S. B. (1997). Psychiatry and the medical model. In S. B. Guze (Ed.), *Washington University adult psychiatry* (pp. 3–14). St. Louis, MO: Mosby.

Bleich, A., Gelkopf, M., & Solomon, Z. (2003). Exposure to terrorism, stress-related mental health symptoms, and coping behaviors among a nationally representative sample in Israel. *Journal of the American Medical Association, 290*, 612–620.

Buysse, D. J. (2008). Chronic insomnia. *American Journal of Psychiatry, 165*, 678–686.

Cloninger, C. R. (2004). *Feeling good: The science of well-being.* New York: Oxford University Press.

Feighner, J. P., Robins, E., Guze, S. B., Woodruff, R. A., Winokur, G., & Munoz, R. (1972). Diagnostic criteria for use in psychiatric research. *Archives of General Psychiatry, 26*, 57–63.

Gabbard, G. O. (2005). Mind, brain and personality disorders. *American Journal of Psychiatry, 162*, 648–655.

Goodwin, D. W., & Guze, S. B. (1996). *Psychiatric diagnosis* (fifth edition). New York: Oxford University Press.

Guze, S. B. (1992). *Why psychiatry is a branch of medicine.* New York: Oxford University Press.

Guze, S. B. (Ed.). (1997). *Washington University adult psychiatry.* St. Louis, MO: Mosby.

Kendell, R., & Jablensky, A. (2003). Distinguishing between the validity and utility of psychiatric diagnoses. *American Journal of Psychiatry, 160*, 4–12.

Kendler, K. S. (2008). Explanatory models for psychiatric illness. *American Journal of Psychiatry, 165*, 695–702.

Lilienfeld, S. O., Lynn, S. J., & Lohr, J. M. (Eds.). (2003). *Science and pseudoscience in clinical psychology.* New York: The Guilford Press.

McHugh, P. R., & Treisman, G. (2007). PTSD: A problematic diagnostic category. *Journal of Anxiety Disorders, 21*, 211–222.

North, C. S., Nixon, S. J., Shariat, S., Mallonee, S., McMillen, J. C., Spitznagel, E. L., et al. (1999). Psychiatric disorders among survivors of the Oklahoma City bombing. *Journal of the American Medical Association, 282*, 755–762.

North, C. S., Osborne, V. A., Vassilenko, M., Kienstra, D. M., Dokucu, M., Hong, B., et al. (2006). Interrater reliability and coding guide for nonpsychotic formal thought disorder. *Perceptual and Motor Skills, 103*, 395–411.

Robins, E., & Guze, S. B. (1970). Establishment of diagnostic validity in psychiatric illness: Its application to schizophrenia. *American Journal of Psychiatry, 126*, 983–987.

Rubin, E. H., & Zorumski, C. F. (Eds.). (2005). *Adult psychiatry* (second edition). Malden, MA: Blackwell Publishing.

Sadock, B. J., & Sadock, V. A. & Ruiz, P. (Eds.). (2009). *Kaplan & Sadock's comprehensive textbook of psychiatry* (ninth edition). Philadelphia: Lippincott Williams & Wilkins.

Spitzer, R. L., Endicott, J., & Robins, E. (1978). Research Diagnostic Criteria: Rationale and reliability. *Archives of General Psychiatry, 35*, 773–782.

Stein, D. J., Seedat, S., Iversen, A., & Wessely, S. (2007). Post-traumatic stress disorder: Medicine and politics. *Lancet, 369*, 139–143.

Zachar, P., & Kendler, K. S. (2007). Psychiatric disorders: A conceptual taxonomy. *American Journal of Psychiatry, 164*, 557–565.

Psychiatric Treatment

Medications

American Psychiatric Association. (2006). *American Psychiatric Association practice guidelines for the treatment of psychiatric disorders. Compendium 2006.* Arlington, VA: American Psychiatric Association.

American Psychiatric Association. (2007). Practice guideline for the treatment of patients with Alzheimer's disease and other dementias (second edition). *American Journal of Psychiatry, 164*(12 Suppl.), 1–56.

American Psychiatric Association. (2007). Practice guideline for the treatment of patients with obsessive-compulsive disorder. *American Journal of Psychiatry, 164*(7 Suppl.), 1–53.

American Psychiatric Association. (2007). Practice guideline for the treatment of patients with substance use disorders (second edition). *American Journal of Psychiatry 164*(4 Suppl.), 1–123.

American Psychiatric Association. (2009). Practice guideline for the treatment of patients with panic disorder (second edition). *American Journal of Psychiatry 166*(2 Suppl.), 1–68.

Barton, O., & Nestler, E. J. (2006). New approaches to antidepressant drug discovery: Beyond monoamines. *Nature Reviews Neuroscience, 7*, 137–151.

Cipriani, A., Furukawa, T. A., Salanti, G., Geddes, J. R., Higgins, J. P. T, Churchill, R., et al. (2009). Comparative efficacy and acceptability of 12 new-generation antidepressants: A multiple-treatments meta-analysis. *Lancet*, *373*, 746–758. Epub ahead of print, Jan 29, DOI: 10.1016/S0140-6736(09)60046-5.

De la Fuente-Fernandez, R., Ruth, T. J., Sossi, V., Schulzer, M., Calne, D. B., & Stoessl, A. J. (2001). Expectation and dopamine release: Mechanism of the placebo effect in Parkinson's disease. *Science*, *293*, 1164–1166.

Jeste, D. V., Blazer, D., Casey, D., Meeks, T., Salzman, C., Schneider, L., et al. (2008). ACNP white paper: Update on use of antipsychotic drugs in elderly persons with dementia. *Neuropsychopharmacology*, *33*, 957–970.

Jones, P. B., Barnes, T. R. E., Davies, L., Dunn, G., Lloyd, H., Hayhurst, K. P., et al. (2006). Randomized controlled trial of the effect on quality of life of second- vs. first-generation antipsychotic drugs in schizophrenia: Cost utility of the latest antipsychotic drugs in schizophrenia study (CUtLASS 1). *Archives of General Psychiatry*, *63*, 1079–1087.

Kindt, M., Soeter, M., & Vervliet, B. (2009). Beyond extinction: Erasing human fear responses and preventing the return of fear. *Nature Neuroscience*, *12*, 256–258.

Kingsbury, S. J., Yi, D., & Simpson, G. M. (2001). Rational and irrational polypharmacy. *Psychiatric Services*, *52*, 1033–1035.

Leon, A. C. (2007). The revised warning for antidepressants and suicidality: Unveiling the black box of statistical analyses. *American Journal of Psychiatry*, *164*, 1786–1789.

Leshner, A. I., Baghdoyan, H. A., Bennett, S. J., Caples, S. M., DeRubeis, R. J., Glynn, R. J., et al. (2005). NIH statement regarding the treatment of insomnia. *Sleep*, *28*, 1049–1057.

Lieberman, J. A. (2006). Comparative effectiveness of antipsychotic drugs. *Archives of General Psychiatry*, *63*, 1069–1072.

Lieberman, J. A., Stroup, T. S., McEvoy, J. P., Swartz, M. S., Rosenheck, R. A., Perkins, D. O., et al. (2005). Effectiveness of antipsychotic drugs in patients with chronic schizophrenia. *New England Journal of Medicine*, *353*, 1209–1223.

Manji, H. K., Moore, G. J., & Chen, G. (1999). Lithium at 50: Have the neuroprotective effects of this unique cation been overlooked? *Biological Psychiatry*, *46*, 929–940.

Mathew, S. J., & Charney, D. S. (2009). Publication bias and the efficacy of antidepressants. *American Journal of Psychiatry*, *166*, 140–145.

Mayberg, H. S., Silva, J. A., Brannan, S. K., Tekell, J. L., Mahurin, R. K., McGinnis, S., et al. (2002). The functional neuroanatomy of the placebo effect. *American Journal of Psychiatry*, *159*, 728–737.

Mazza, M., Pomponi, M., Janiri, L., Bria, P., & Mazza, S. (2007). Omega-3 fatty acids and antioxidants in neurological and psychiatric diseases: An overview. *Progress in Neuro-psychopharmacology and Biological Psychiatry*, *31*, 12–26.

Rosenheck, R. A. (2006). Outcomes, cost and policy caution. *Archives of General Psychiatry*, *63*, 1074–1076.

Rosenheck, R. A., Leslie, D. L., Sindelar, J., Miller, E. A., Lin, H., Stroup, T. S., et al. (2006). Cost-effectiveness of second-generation antipsychotics and perphenazine in a randomized trial of treatment for chronic schizophrenia. *American Journal of Psychiatry*, *163*, 2080–2089.

Rubin, E. H., & Zorumski, C. F. (Eds.). (2005). *Adult psychiatry* (second edition). Malden, MA: Blackwell Publishing.

Rush, A. J. (2007). STAR*D: What have we learned? *American Journal of Psychiatry*, *164*, 201–204.

Rush, A. J., Trivedi, M. H., Wisniewski, S. R., Nierenberg, A. A., Stewart, J. W., Warden, D., et al. (2006). Acute and longer-term outcomes in depressed outpatients requiring one of several treatment steps: A STAR*D report. *American Journal of Psychiatry*, *163*, 1905–1917.

Rush, A. J., Trivedi, M. H., Wisniewski, S. R., Stewart, J. W., Nierenberg, A. A., Thase, M. E., et al. (2006). Buproprion-SR, sertraline or venlafaxine-XR after failure of SSRIs for depression. *New England Journal of Medicine*, *354*, 1231–1242.

Sadock, B. J., Sadock, V. A. & Ruiz, P. (Eds.). (2009). *Kaplan & Sadock's comprehensive textbook of psychiatry* (ninth edition). Philadelphia: Lippincott Williams & Wilkins.

Schatzberg, A. F., & Nemeroff, C. B. (Eds.). (2006). *Essentials of clinical psychopharmacology* (second edition). Washington, DC: American Psychiatric Publishing.

Spanagel, R., & Kiefer, F. (2008). Drugs for relapse prevention of alcoholism: Ten years of progress. *Trends in Pharmacological Sciences*, *29*, 109–115.

Trivedi, M. H., Fava, M., Wisniewski, S. R., Thase, M. E., Quitkin, F., Warden, D., et al. (2006). Medication augmentation after the failure of SSRIs for depression. *New England Journal of Medicine*, *354*, 1243–1252.

Turner, E. H., Matthews, N. M., Linardatos, E., Tell, R. A., & Rosenthal, R. (2008). Selective publication of antidepressant trials and its influence on apparent efficacy. *New England Journal of Medicine, 358*, 252–260.

Electroconvulsive Therapy and Brain Stimulation

Abrams, R. (2002). *Electroconvulsive therapy* (fourth edition). New York: Oxford University Press.
Dukakis, K., & Tye, L. (2006). *Shock: The healing power of electroconvulsive therapy.* New York: Avery.
George, M. S., Lisanby, S. H., & Sackeim, H. A. (1999). Transcranial magnetic stimulation: Applications in neuropsychiatry. *Archives of General Psychiatry, 56*, 300–311.
Gershon, A. A., Dannon, P. N., & Grunhaus, L. (2003). Transcranial magnetic stimulation in the treatment of depression. *American Journal of Psychiatry, 160*, 835–845.
Hardesty, D. E., & Sackeim, H. A. (2007). Deep brain stimulation in movement and psychiatric disorders. *Biological Psychiatry, 61*, 831–835.
Janicak, P. G., Dowd, S. M., Strong, M. J., Alam, D., & Beedle, D. (2005). The potential role of repetitive transcranial magnetic stimulation in treating severe depression. *Psychiatric Annals, 35*, 138–145.
Mashour, G. A., Walker, E. E., & Martuza, R. L. (2005). Psychosurgery: Past, present and future. *Brain Research Reviews, 48*, 409–419.
Mayberg, H. S., Lozano, A. M., Voon, V., McNeely, H. E., Seminowicz, D., Hamani, C., et al. (2005). Deep brain stimulation for treatment-resistant depression. *Neuron, 45*, 651–660.
Nemeroff, C. B., Mayberg, H. S., Krahl, S. E., McNamara, J., Frazer, A., Henry, T. R., et al. (2006). VNS therapy in treatment-resistant depression: Clinical evidence and putative neurobiological mechanisms. *Neuropsychopharmacology, 31*, 1345–1355.
Sackeim, H. A., Prudic, J., Devanand, D. P., Nobler, M. S., Lisanby, S. H., Peyser, S., et al. (2000). A prospective, randomized, double-blind comparison of bilateral and right unilateral electroconvulsive therapy at different stimulus intensities. *Archives of General Psychiatry, 57*, 425–434.
Sackeim, H. A., Prudic, J., Fuller, R., Keilp, J., Lavori, P. W., & Olfson, M. (2007). The cognitive effects of electroconvulsive therapy in community settings. *Neuropsychopharmacology, 32*, 244–254.
Shuchman, M. (2007). Approving the vagus-nerve stimulator for depression. *New England Journal of Medicine, 356*, 1604–1607.
Wichmann, T., & DeLong, M. R. (2006). Deep brain stimulation for neurologic and neuropsychiatric disorders. *Neuron, 52*, 197–204.
Zorumski, C. F., de Erausquin, G., Dokucu, M., Svrakic, D., Garcia, K., & Jarvis, M. (2008). Brain stimulation and the treatment of refractory psychiatric disorders. *Missouri Medicine, 105*, 57–61.

Psychotherapies and Lifestyle

Axelrod, R. (1984). *The evolution of cooperation.* Cambridge, MA: Basic Books.
Barabási, A.-L. (2002). *Linked: The new science of networks.* Cambridge, MA: Perseus Publishing.
Bateman, A., & Fonagy, P. (2008). Eight-year follow-up of patients treated for borderline personality disorder: Mentalization-based treatment versus treatment as usual. *American Journal of Psychiatry, 165*, 631–638.
Beauregard, M. (2007). Mind does really matter: Evidence from neuroimaging studies of emotional self-regulation, psychotherapy and placebo effect. *Progress in Neurobiology, 81*, 218–236.
Burns, D. D. (1980). *Feeling good: The new mood therapy.* New York: William Morrow & Co.
Charney, D. S. (2004). Psychobiological mechanisms of resilience and vulnerability: Implications for successful adaptation to extreme stress. *American Journal of Psychiatry, 161*, 195–216.
Cloninger, C. R. (2004). *Feeling good: The science of well-being.* New York: Oxford University Press.
Fulgham, R. (1996). *All I really need to know I learned in kindergarten: Uncommon thoughts on common things.* New York: Fawcett Columbine.
Gabbard, G. O., & Kay, J. (2001). The fate of integrated treatment: Whatever happened to the biopsychosocial psychiatrist? *American Journal of Psychiatry, 158*, 1956–1963.
Guze, S.B. (1988). Psychotherapy and the etiology of psychiatric disorders. *Psychiatric Developments, 6*, 183–193.
Keller, M. B., McCullough, J. P., Klein, D. N., Arnow, B., Dunner, D. L., Gelenberg, A. J., et al. (2000). A comparison of nefazodone, the cognitive behavioral analysis system of psychotherapy and

their combination for the treatment of chronic depression. *New England Journal of Medicine,* *342,* 1462–1470.

Kennedy, S. H., Konarski, J. Z., Segal, Z. V., Lau, M. A., Bieling, P. J., McIntyre, R. S., et al. (2007). Differences in brain glucose metabolism between responders to CBT and venlafaxine in a 16-week randomized controlled trial. *American Journal of Psychiatry, 164,* 778–788.

Lilienfeld, S. O., Lynn, S. J., & Lohr, J. M. (Eds.). (2003). *Science and pseudoscience in clinical psychology.* New York: The Guilford Press.

Linehan, M. M. (1987). Dialectical behavior therapy for borderline personality disorder. *Bulletin of the Menninger Clinic, 51,* 261–276.

Linehan, M. M., Armstrong, H. E., Suarez, A., Allmon, D., & Heard, H. L. (1991). Cognitive-behavioral treatment of chronically parasuicidal borderline patients. *Archives of General Psychiatry, 48,* 1060–1064.

Nemeroff, C. B., Heim, C. M., Thase, M. E., Klein, D. N., Rush, A. J., Schatzberg, A. F., et al. (2003). Differential responses to psychotherapy versus pharmacotherapy in patients with chronic forms of major depression and childhood trauma. *Proceedings of the National Academy of Sciences (USA), 100,* 14293–14296.

Paulos, M. P. (2007). Decision making dysfunctions in psychiatry: Altered homeostatic processing? *Science, 318,* 602–606.

Rubin, E. H., & Zorumski, C. F. (Eds.). (2005). *Adult psychiatry* (second edition). Malden, MA: Blackwell Publishing.

Sadock, B. J., Sadock, V. A. & Ruiz, P. (Eds.). (2009). *Kaplan & Sadock's comprehensive textbook of psychiatry* (ninth edition). Philadelphia: Lippincott Williams & Wilkins.

Seligman, M. E. P., Rashid, T., & Parks, A. C. (2006). Positive psychotherapy. *American Psychologist, 61,* 772–788.

Vaillant, G. E. (2003). Mental health. *American Journal of Psychiatry, 160,* 1373–1384.

Vaillant, G. E., DiRago, A. C., & Mukamal, K. (2006). Natural history of male psychological health, XV: Retirement satisfaction. *American Journal of Psychiatry, 163,* 682–688.

Verghese, J., Lipton, R. B., Katz, M. J., Hall, C. B., Derby, C. A., Kuslansky, G., et al. (2003). Leisure activities and the risk of dementia in the elderly. *New England Journal of Medicine, 348,* 2508–2516.

Weissman, M. M., Markowitz, J. C., & Klerman, G. L. (2000). *Comprehensive guide to interpersonal therapy.* New York: Basic Books.

Willis, S. L., Tennstedt. D. L., Marsiske, M., Ball, K., Elias, J., Koepke, K. M., et al. (2006). Long-term effects of cognitive training on everyday functional outcomes in older adults. *Journal of the American Medical Association, 296,* 2805–2814.

Wilson, R. S., Medes de Leon, C. F., Barnes, L. L., Schneider, J. A., Bienias, J. L., Evans, D. A., et al. (2002). Participation in cognitively stimulating activities and risk of incident Alzheimer disease. *Journal of the American Medical Association, 287,* 742–748.

Witte, A. V., Fobker, M., Gellner, R., Knecht, S., & Flöel, A. (2009). Caloric restriction improves memory in elderly humans. *Proceedings of the National Academy of Sciences (USA), 106,* 1255–1260.

Genetics and Psychiatry

Attia, J., Ioannidis, J. P. A., Thakkinstian, A., McEvoy, M., Scott, R. J., Minelli, C., et al. (2009). How to use an article about genetic association. A. Background concepts. *Journal of the American Medical Association, 301,* 74–81.

Caspi, A., McClay, J., Moffitt, T. E., Mill, J., Martin, J., Craig, I. W., et al. (2002). Role of genotype in the cycle of violence in maltreated children. *Science, 297,* 851–854.

Caspi, A., & Moffitt, T. E. (2006). Gene–environment interactions in psychiatry: Joining forces with neuroscience. *Nature Reviews Neuroscience, 7,* 583–590.

Caspi, A., Sugden, K., Moffitt, T. E., Taylor, A., Craig, I. W., Harrington, H., et al. (2003). Influence of life stress on depression: Moderation by a polymorphism in the 5-HTT gene. *Science, 301,* 386–389.

Feinberg, A. P. (2008). Epigenetics at the epicenter of modern medicine. *Journal of the American Medical Association, 299,* 1345–1350.

Gottesman, I. I., & Gould, T. D. (2003). The endophenotype concept in psychiatry: Etymology and strategic intentions. *American Journal of Psychiatry, 160,* 636–645.

Kendler, K. S. (2005). Psychiatric genetics: A methodologic critique. *American Journal of Psychiatry,* *162*, 3–11.

Kendler, K. S. (2006). Reflections on the relationship between psychiatric genetics and psychiatric nosology. *American Journal of Psychiatry, 163,* 1138–1146.

Kendler, K. S., & Baker, J. H. (2007). Genetic influences on measures of the environment: A systematic review. *Psychological Medicine, 37,* 615–626.

McGowan, P. O., Sasaki, A., D'Alessio, A. C., Dymov, S., Labonté, B., Szyf, M., et al. (2009). Epigenetic regulation of the glucocorticoid receptor in human brain associates with childhood abuse. *Nature Neuroscience, 12,* 342–348.

Merikangas, K. (2001). Genetic epidemiology: Bringing genetics to the population. *Acta Psychiatrica Scandinavica, 104,* 1–11.

Merikangas, K. R., & Risch, N. (2003). Will the genomics revolution revolutionize psychiatry? *American Journal of Psychiatry, 160,* 625–635.

Munafò, M. R., Durrant, C., Lewis, G., & Flint, J. (2009). Gene x environment interactions at the serotonin transporter locus. *Biological Psychiatry, 65,* 211–219.

Ridley, M. (2003). *Nature via nurture: Genes, experience, and what makes us human.* New York: HarperCollins Publishers.

Walsh, T., McClellan, J. M., McCarthy, S. E., Addington, A. M., Pierce, S. B., Cooper, G. M., et al. (2008). Rare structural variants disrupt multiple genes in neurodevelopmental pathways in schizophrenia. *Science, 320,* 539–543.

Zorumski, C. F., & Rubin, E. H. (Eds.). (2005). *Psychopathology in the genome and neuroscience era.* Washington, DC: American Psychiatric Publishing.

Brain Mechanisms

General

Andreasen, N. C. (2005). *The creating brain: The neuroscience of genius.*, New York: Dana Press.

Axelrod, R. (1984). *The evolution of cooperation.* Cambridge, MA: Basic Books.

Barabási, A.-L. (2002). *Linked: The new science of networks.* Cambridge, MA: Perseus Publishing.

Damasio, A. (1999). *The feeling of what happens: Body and emotion in the making of consciousness.* San Diego, CA: Harcourt.

Edelman, G. M. (2004). *Wider than the sky: The phenomenal gift of consciousness.* New Haven, CT: Yale University Press.

Gazzaniga, M. S. (2005). *The ethical brain: The science of our moral dilemmas.* New York: Dana Press.

Goldberg, E. (2001). *The executive brain: Frontal lobes and the civilized mind.* New York: Oxford University Press.

Hawkins, J. (with Blakeslee, S.). (2004). *On intelligence.* New York: Times Books.

Kandel, E. R. (2006). *In search of memory: The emergence of a new science of mind.* New York: WW Norton & Company.

LeDoux, J. (2002). *Synaptic self: How our brains become who we are.* New York: Viking Press.

Linden, D. J. (2007). *The accidental mind: How brain evolution has given us love, memory, dreams, and God.* Cambridge, MA: Belknap Press.

Minsky, M. (2006). *The emotion machine: Commonsense thinking, artificial intelligence, and the future of the human mind.* New York: Simon & Schuster.

Montague, R. (2006). *Why choose this book? How we make decisions.* New York: Dutton Press.

Panksepp, J. (2004). *Affective neuroscience: The foundations of human and animal emotions.* New York: Oxford University Press.

Quartz, S. R., & Sejnowski, T. J. (2002). *Liars, lovers and heroes: What the new brain science reveals about how we become who we are.* New York: William Morrow.

Ramachandran, V. S. (2004). *A brief tour of human consciousness: From impostor poodles to purple numbers.* New York: Pi Press.

Ramachandran, V. S., & Blakeslee, S. (1998). *Phantoms in the brain: Probing the mysteries of the human mind.* New York: William Morrow.

Ridley, M. (2003). *Nature via nurture: Genes, experience, and what makes us human.* New York: HarperCollins Publishers.

Schacter, D. L. (2001). *The seven sins of memory: How the mind forgets and remembers.* Boston: Houghton Mifflin.

Watts, D. J. (2003). *Six degrees: The science of a connected age.* New York: WW Norton & Company.

Zorumski, C. F., & Rubin, E. H. (Eds.). (2005). *Psychopathology in the genome and neuroscience era.* Washington, DC: American Psychiatric Publishing.

Illness-Related Brain Changes

Benes, F. M. (2007). Searching for unique endophenotypes for schizophrenia and bipolar disorder within neural circuits and their molecular regulatory mechanisms. *Schizophrenia Bulletin, 33,* 932–936.

Botteron, K. N., Raichle, M. E., Drevets, W. C., Heath, A. C., & Todd, R. D. (2002). Volumetric reduction in left subgenual prefrontal cortex in early onset depression. *Biological Psychiatry, 51,* 342–344.

Bremner, J. D., Narayan, M., Anderson, E. R., Staib, L. H., Miller, H. L., & Charney, D. S. (2000). Hippocampal volume reduction in major depression. *American Journal of Psychiatry, 157,* 115–118.

Drevets, W. C. (1999). Prefrontal cortical-amygdalar metabolism in major depression. *Annals of the New York Academy of Sciences, 877,* 614–637.

Drevets, W. C., Price, J. L., Simpson, J. R., Todd, R. D., Reich, T., Vannier, M., et al. (1997). Subgenual prefrontal cortex abnormalities in mood disorders. *Nature, 386,* 824–827.

Feinberg, A. P. (2008). Epigenetics at the epicenter of modern medicine. *Journal of the American Medical Association, 299,* 1345–1350.

Gilbertson, M. W., Shenton, M. E., Ciszewski, A., Kasai, K., Lasko, N. B., Orr, S. P., et al (2002). Smaller hippocampal volume predicts pathologic vulnerability to psychological trauma. *Nature Neuroscience, 5,* 1242–1247.

Harrison, P. J. (2002). The neuropathology of primary mood disorder. *Brain, 7,* 1428–1449.

Hyman, S. E., & Malenka, R. C. (2001). Addiction and the brain: The neurobiology of compulsion and its persistence. *Nature Reviews Neuroscience, 2,* 695–703.

Johansen-Berg, H., Gutman, D. A., Behrens, T. E. J., Matthews, P. M., Rushworth, M. F. S., Katz, E., et al. (2008). Anatomical connectivity of the subgenual cingulate region targeted with deep brain stimulation for treatment-resistant depression. *Cerebral Cortex, 18,* 1374–1383.

Kapur, S. (2003). Psychosis as a state of aberrant salience: A framework linking biology, phenomenology and pharmacology in schizophrenia. *American Journal of Psychiatry, 160,* 13–23.

King-Casas, B., Sharp, C., Lomax-Bream, L., Lohrenz, T., Fonagy, P., & Montague, P.R. (2008). The rupture and repair of cooperation in borderline personality disorder. *Science, 321,* 806–810.

Lewis, D. A., & Hashimoto, T. (2007). Deciphering the disease process of schizophrenia: The contribution of cortical GABA neurons. *International Review of Neurobiology, 78,* 109–131.

Manji, H., Drevets, W. C., & Charney, D. S. (2001). The cellular neurobiology of depression. *Nature Medicine, 7,* 541–547.

Mathis, C. A., Klunk, W. E., Price, J. C., & DeKosky, S. T. (2005). Imaging technology for neurodegenerative diseases: Progress toward detection of specific pathologies. *Archives of Neurology, 62,* 196–200.

McEwen, B. S. (2007). Physiology and neurobiology of stress and adaptation: Central role of the brain. *Physiological Reviews, 87,* 873–904.

Morris, J. C., Galvin, J. E., & Holtzman, D. M. (Eds.). (2006). *Handbook of dementing illnesses* (second edition). New York: Taylor & Francis.

Olney, J. W., Young, C., Wozniak, D. F., Jevtovic-Todorovic, V., & Ikonomidou, C. (2004). Do pediatric drugs cause developing neurons to commit suicide? *Trends in Pharmacological Sciences, 25,* 135–139.

Ongur, D., Drevets, W. C., & Price, J. L. (1998). Glial reduction in the subgenual prefrontal cortex in mood disorders. *Proceedings of the National Academy of Sciences (USA), 27,* 13290–13295.

Sapolsky, R. M. (2000). Glucocorticoids and hippocampal atrophy in neuropsychiatric disorders. *Archives of General Psychiatry, 57,* 925–935.

Seminowicz, D. A., Mayberg, H. S., McIntosh, A. R., Goldapple, K., Kennedy, S., Segal, Z., et al. (2004). Limbic-frontal circuitry in major depression: A path modeling metanalysis. *Neuroimage, 22,* 409–418.

Sheline, Y., Sanghavi, M., Mintun, M., & Gado, M. (1999). Depression duration but not age predicts hippocampal volume loss in women with recurrent major depression. *Journal of Neuroscience, 19,* 5034–5043.

Sheline, Y., Wang, P., Gado, M., Csernansky, J., & Vannier, M. (1996). Hippocampal atrophy in recurrent major depression. *Proceedings of the National Academy of Sciences (USA), 93,* 3908–3913.

Shulman, R. G. (2001). Functional imaging studies: Linking mind and basic neuroscience. *American Journal of Psychiatry, 158,* 11–20.

Vythilingam, M., Heim, C., Newport, J., Miller, A. H., Anderson, E., Bronen, R., et al. (2002). Childhood trauma associated with smaller hippocampal volume in women with major depression. *American Journal of Psychiatry, 159,* 2072–2080.

Emotions, Plasticity, and Neurogenesis

Airan, R. D., Meltzer, L. A., Roy, M., Gong, Y., Chen, H., & Deisseroth, K. (2007). High-speed imaging reveals neurophysiological links to behavior in an animal model of depression. *Science, 317,* 819–823.

Alcaro, A., Huber, R., & Panksepp, J. (2007). Behavioral functions of the mesolimbic dopaminergic system: An affective neuroethological perspective. *Brain Research Reviews, 56,* 283–321.

Becker, S., & Wojtowicz, J. M. (2006). A model of hippocampal neurogenesis in memory and mood disorders. *Trends in Cognitive Sciences, 11,* 70–76.

Burgdorf, J., & Panksepp, J. (2006). The neurobiology of positive emotion. *Neuroscience and Biobehavioral Reviews, 30,* 173–187.

Dosenbach, N. U. F., Fair, D. A., Cohen, A. L., Schlagger, L. B., & Petersen, S. E. (2008). A dual-networks architecture of top-down control. *Trends in Cognitive Sciences, 12,* 99–105.

Feinberg, A. P. (2008). Epigenetics at the epicenter of modern medicine. *Journal of the American Medical Association, 299,* 1345–1350.

Kauer, J. A., & Malenka, R. C. (2007). Synaptic plasticity and addiction. *Nature Reviews Neuroscience, 8,* 844–858.

Kempermann, G. (2008). The neurogenic reserve hypothesis: What is adult hippocampal neurogenesis good for? *Trends in Neurosciences, 31,* 163–169.

Lowenstein, G., Rick, S., & Cohen, J. D. (2008). Neuroeconomics. *Annual Review of Psychology, 59,* 647–672.

McClung, C. A., & Nestler, E. J. (2008). Neuroplasticity mediated by altered gene expression. *Neuropsychopharmacology, 33,* 3–17.

Meaney, M. J., & Szyf, M. (2005). Maternal care as a model for experience-dependent chromatin plasticity? *Trends in Neurosciences, 28,* 456–463.

Montague, P. R., King-Casas, B., & Cohen, J. D. (2006). Imaging valuation models in human choice. *Annual Review of Neuroscience, 29,* 417–448.

Panksepp, J. (2006). Emotional endophenotypes in evolutionary psychiatry. *Progress in Neuropsychopharmacology and Biological Psychiatry, 30,* 774–784.

Pittenger, C., & Duman, R. S. (2008). Stress, depression and neuroplasticity: A convergence of mechanisms. *Neuropsychopharmacology, 33,* 88–109.

Raichle, M. E., & Snyder, A. Z. (2007). A default mode of brain function: A brief history of an evolving idea. *Neuroimage, 37,* 1083–1090.

Sahay, A., & Hen, R. (2007). Adult hippocampal neurogenesis in depression. *Nature Neuroscience, 10,* 1110–1115.

Santarelli, L., Saxe, M., Gross, C., Surget, A., Battaglia, F., Dulawa, S., et al. (2003). Requirement of hippocampal neurogenesis for the behavioral effects of antidepressants. *Science, 301,* 805–809.

Schloss, P., & Henn, F. A. (2004) New insights into the mechanisms of antidepressant therapy. *Pharmacology and Therapeutics, 102,* 47–60.

Sheline, Y. I., Barch, D. M., Price, J. L., Rundle, M. M., Vaishnavi, S. N., Snyder, A. Z., et al. (2009). The default mode network and self-referential processes in depression. *Proceedings of the National Academy of Sciences (USA), 106,* 1942–1947.

Song, H., Stevens, C. F., & Gage, F. H. (2002). Neural stem cells from adult hippocampus develop essential properties of functional CNS neurons. *Nature Neuroscience, 5,* 438–445.

Warren-Schmidt, J. L., & Duman, R. S. (2006). Hippocampal neurogenesis: Opposing effects of stress and antidepressant treatment. *Hippocampus, 16,* 239–249.

Whitfield-Gabrieli, S., Thermenos, H. W., Milanovic, S., Tsuang, M. T., Faraone, S. V., McCarley, R. W., et al. (2009). Hyperactivity and hyperconnectivity of the default network in schizophrenia and in first-degree relatives of persons with schizophrenia. *Proceedings of the National Academy of Sciences (USA)*, *106*, 1279–1284.

Zorumski, C. F. (2005). Neurobiology, neurogenesis and the pathology of psychopathology. In C.F. Zorumski & E. H. Rubin (Eds.), *Psychopathology in the genome and neuroscience era* (pp. 175–187), Washington, DC: American Psychiatric Publishing.

Psychiatry and Public Health

Compton, W. M., Grant, B. F., Colliver, J. D., Glantz, M. D., & Stinson, F. S. (2004). Prevalence of marijuana use disorders in the United States: 1991–1992 and 2001–2002. *Journal of the American Medical Association*, *291*, 114–121.

Demyttenaere, K., Bruffaerts, R., Posada-Villa, J., Gasquet, I., Kovess, V., Lepine, J. P., et al. (2004). Prevalence, severity, and unmet need for treatment of mental disorders in the World Health Organization World Mental Health Surveys. *Journal of the American Medical Association*, *291*, 2581–2590.

Fiore, M. C., Jaén, C. R., Baker, T. B., Bailey, W. C., Benowitz, N. L., Curry, S. J., et al. (2008). *Treating tobacco use and dependence: 2008 update. Clinical Practice Guideline*. Rockville, MD: U.S. Department of Health and Human Services. Public Health Service.

Gilbody, S., Bower, P., Fletcher, J., Richards, D., & Sutton, A. J. (2006). Collaborative care for depression: A cumulative meta-analysis and review of longer-term outcomes. *Archives of Internal Medicine*, *166*, 2314–2321.

Goldsmith, S. K., Pellman, T. C., Kleinman, A. M., & Bunney, W. E. (Eds.) (2002). *Reducing suicide: A national imperative*. Washington, DC: National Academies Press.

Iglehart, J. K. (2004). The mental health maze and the call for transformation. *New England Journal of Medicine*, *350*, 507–514.

Insel, T. R. (2009). Translating scientific opportunity into public health impact: A strategic plan for research on mental illness. *Archives of General Psychiatry*, *66*, 128–133.

Katon, W., & Unützer, J. (2006). Collaborative care models for depression: Time to move from evidence to practice. *Archives of Internal Medicine*, *166*, 2304–2306.

Kessler, R. C., Berglund, P., Demler, O., Jin, R., Merikangas, K.R., & Walters, E.E. (2005). Lifetime prevalence and age-of-onset distributions of DSM-IV disorders in the National Comorbidity Survey replication. *Archives of General Psychiatry*, *62*, 593–602.

Kessler, R. C., Demler, O., Frank, R. G., Olfson, M., Pincus, H. A., Walters, E. E., et al. (2005). Prevalence and treatment of mental disorders, 1990 to 2003. *New England Journal of Medicine*, *352*, 2515–2523.

Kessler, R. C., Heeringa, S., Lakoma, M. D., Petukhova, M., Rupp, A. E., Schoenbaum, M., et al. (2008). Individual and societal effects of mental disorders on earnings in the United States: Results from the National Comorbidity Survey Replication. *American Journal of Psychiatry*, *165*, 703–711.

Merikangas, K. R., Ames, M., Cui, L., Stang, P. E., Ustun, T. B., Von Korff, M., et al. (2007). The impact of comorbidity of mental and physical conditions on role disability in the US adult household population. *Archives of General Psychiatry*, *64*, 1180–1188.

Mokdad, A. H., Marks, J. S., Stroup, D. F., & Gerberding, J. E. (2004). Actual causes of death in the United States, 2000. *Journal of the American Medical Association*, *291*, 1238–1245.

Moussavi, S., Chatterji, S., Verdes, E., Tandon, A., Patel, V., & Ustun, B. (2007). Depression, chronic diseases, and decrements in health: Results from the World Health Surveys. *Lancet*, *370*, 851–858.

Newcomer, J. W., & Hennekens, C. H. (2007). Severe mental illness and risk of cardiovascular disease. *Journal of the American Medical Association*, *298*, 1794–1796.

Prince, M., Patel, V., Saxena, S., Maj, M., Maselko, J., Phillips, M. R., et al. (2007). No health without mental health. *Lancet*, *370*, 859–877.

Saha, S., Chant, D., & McGrath, J. (2007). A systematic review of mortality in schizophrenia. *Archives of General Psychiatry*, *64*, 1123–1131.

Saitz, R. (2005). Unhealthy alcohol use. *New England Journal of Medicine*, *352*, 596–607.

Stewart, M. F., Ricci, J. A., Chee, E., Hahn, S. R., & Morganstein, D. (2003). Cost of lost productive work time among US workers with depression. *Journal of the American Medical Association*, *289*, 3135–3144.

Ustun, T. B., Ayuso-Mateos, J. L., Chatterji, S., Mathers, C., & Murray, C. J. L. (2004). Global burden of depressive disorders in the year 2000. *British Journal of Psychiatry, 184,* 386–392.

Trends in Psychiatry

Angell, M. (2004). *The truth about the drug companies: How they deceive us and what to do about it.* New York: Random House.

Bok, D. (2003). *Universities in the marketplace: The commercialization of higher education.* Princeton, NJ: Princeton University Press.

Cowan, W. M., & Kandel, E. R. (2001). Prospects for neurology and psychiatry. *Journal of the American Medical Association, 285,* 594–600.

Hyman, S. E. (2007). Can neuroscience be integrated into the DSM-V? *Nature Reviews Neuroscience, 8,* 725–732.

Kassirer, J. P. (2005). *On the take: How medicine's complicity with big business can endanger your health.* New York: Oxford University Press.

Meyer, R. E., & McLaughlin, C. J. (Eds.). (1998). *Between mind, brain, and managed care: The now and future world of academic psychiatry.* Washington, DC: American Psychiatric Press.

Rubin, E. H. (2005). The complexities of individual financial conflicts of interest. *Neuropsychopharmacology, 30,* 1–6.

Rubin, E. H., & Zorumski, C. F. (2003). The impact of scientific advances on the future of psychiatric education. *Academic Medicine, 78,* 351–354.

Rubin, E. H., & Zorumski, C. F. (2005). The influence of scientific advances, workforce issues and educational trends on psychiatric training. In C. F. Zorumski & E. H. Rubin (Eds.), *Psychopathology in the genome and neuroscience era* (pp. 191–202). Washington, DC: American Psychiatric Publishing.

Wazana, A. (2000). Physicians and the pharmaceutical industry: Is a gift ever just a gift? *Journal of the American Medical Association, 283,* 373–380.

Zorumski, C. F., & Rubin, E. H. (Eds.). (2005). *Psychopathology in the genome and neuroscience era.* Washington, DC: American Psychiatric Publishing.

Index